Lesbian, Gay, Bisexual, and Transgender Dermatology

Editors

LAUREN MESHKOV BONATI

JARED JAGDEO

DERMATOLOGIC CLINICS

www.derm.theclinics.com

Consulting Editor

BRUCE H. THIERS

April 2020 • Volume 38 • Number 2

ELSEVIER

1600 John F. Kennedy Boulevard ● Suite 1800 ● Philadelphia, Pennsylvania, 19103-2899

http://www.theclinics.com

DERMATOLOGIC CLINICS Volume 38, Number 2
April 2020 ISSN 0733-8635, ISBN-13: 978-0-323-71127-2

Editor: Lauren Boyle
Developmental Editor: Laura Kavanaugh

Dermatologic Clinics (ISSN 0733-8635) is published quarterly by Elsevier Inc., 360 Park Avenue South, New York, NY 10010-1710. Months of publication are January, April, July, and October. Business and editorial offices: 1600 John F. Kennedy Blvd., Suite 1800, Philadelphia, PA 19103-2899. Customer service office: 11830 Westline Drive, St. Louis, MO 63146. Periodicals postage paid at New York, NY, and additional mailing offices. Subscription prices are USD 408.00 per year for US individuals, USD 780.00 per year for US institutions, USD 456.00 per year for Canadian individuals, USD 952.00 per year for Canadian institutions, USD 510.00 per year for international individuals, USD 952.00 per year for international institutions, USD 100.00 per year for US students/residents, USD 100.00 per year for Canadian students/residents, and USD 240 per year for international students/residents. International air speed delivery is included in all *Clinics* subscription prices. All prices are subject to change without notice. **POSTMASTER:** Send address changes to *Dermatologic Clinics*, Elsevier Health Sciences Division, Subscription Customer Service, 3251 Riverport Lane, Maryland Heights, MO 63043. **Customer Service: 1-800-654-2452 (U.S. and Canada); 314-447-8871 (outside U.S. and Canada). Fax: 314-447-8029. E-mail: journalscustomerservice-usa@elsevier.com (for print support); journalsonlinesupport-usa@elsevier.com (for online support).**

Reprints. For copies of 100 or more, of articles in this publication, please contact the Commercial Reprints Department, Elsevier Inc., 360 Park Avenue South, New York, New York 10010-1710. Tel.: 212-633-3874; Fax: 212-633-3820; Email: reprints@elsevier.com.

The *Dermatologic Clinics* is covered in *MEDLINE/PubMed (Index Medicus)*, *Current Contents/Clinical Medicine*, *Excerpta Medica, Chemical Abstracts,* and *ISI/BIOMED*.

Contributors

CONSULTING EDITOR

BRUCE H. THIERS, MD
Professor and Chairman Emeritus, Department
of Dermatology and Dermatologic Surgery,
Medical University of South Carolina,
Charleston, South Carolina

EDITORS

LAUREN MESHKOV BONATI, MD, FAAD
Director of Dermatologic and Cosmetic Laser
Surgery, Mountain Dermatology Specialists,
Edwards, Colorado

JARED JAGDEO, MD, FAAD
Associate Professor of Dermatology, Director
of the Center for Photomedicine, Director of the
Laser, Aesthetics, and Body Institute, SUNY
Downstate Medical Center, Brooklyn, New
York

AUTHORS

ANDRE ALCON, MD
Resident Physician, Division of Plastic and
Reconstructive Surgery, University of
California, San Francisco, San Francisco,
California

ERICA ARNOLD, BS
University of Utah School of Medicine,
Salt Lake City, Utah, Spring Street
Dermatology, New York University, New York,
New York

SARAH TUTTLETON ARRON, MD, PhD
Associate Professor of Dermatology,
University of California, San Francisco,
San Francisco, California

BRITTANY BUHALOG, MD
Fellow Physician, Department of Dermatologic
Surgery, University of California, San
Francisco, San Francisco, California

YUNYOUNG C. CHANG, MD
Union Square Laser Dermatology, New York,
New York

STEVEN DAVELUY, MD
Associate Professor, Department of
Dermatology, Wayne State University School
of Medicine, Detroit, Michigan

NIKHIL DHINGRA, MD
Clinical Instructor, Department of
Dermatology, Icahn School of Medicine at
Mount Sinai, Spring Street Dermatology, New
York University, New York, New York

AMANDA E. DILGER, MD
AAFPRS Fellow, Facial Plastic and
Reconstructive Surgery, Roseville, California

JOSEPH W. FAKHOURY, BS
Medical Student, Department of Dermatology,
Wayne State University School of Medicine,
Detroit, Michigan

WILLIAM HOFFMAN, MD
Professor and Chief, Division of Plastic and
Reconstructive Surgery, University of
California, San Francisco, San Francisco,
California

JUSTIN L. JIA, BS
Department of Dermatology, Stanford
University School of Medicine, Redwood City,
California

BENJAMIN KAHN, MD
Department of Dermatology, Emory University
School of Medicine, Atlanta, Georgia

KENNETH A. KATZ, MD, MSc, MSCE
Department of Dermatology, Kaiser
Permanente, San Francisco, California

MARYIA KAZLOUSKAYA, BA
CUNY Queens College, Queens, New York

VIKTORYIA KAZLOUSKAYA, MD, PhD
SUNY Downstate Medical Center, Brooklyn,
New York

ESTHER A. KIM, MD, FACS
Assistant Professor, Division of Plastic and
Reconstructive Surgery, Chief of UCSF
Transgender Surgery, University of California,
San Francisco, San Francisco, California

PHILIP DANIEL KNOTT, MD, FACS
Professor and Director, Section of Facial Plastic
Surgery, Fellowship Director, Facial Plastic and
Reconstructive Surgery, Department of
Otolaryngology–Head and Neck Surgery, UCSF
Medical Center, San Francisco, California

CARRIE L. KOVARIK, MD
Associate Professor, Department of
Dermatology, Perelman School of Medicine,
University of Pennsylvania, Philadelphia,
Pennsylvania

YI CHUN LAI, MD, MPH
SUNY Downstate Medical Center, Brooklyn,
New York

BAOCHAU LY, BS
Department of Dermatology, Emory University
School of Medicine, Atlanta, Georgia

JENNIFER L. MacGREGOR, MD
Union Square Laser Dermatology, New York,
New York

MATTHEW MANSH, MD
Assistant Professor, Department of
Dermatology, University of Minnesota School
of Medicine, Minneapolis, Minnesota

JULIA L. MARCUS, PhD, MPH
Department of Population Medicine, Harvard
Medical School, Harvard Pilgrim Health Care
Institute, Boston, Massachusetts

DUSTIN H. MARKS, BS
Department of Dermatology, Massachusetts
General Hospital, Boston, Massachusetts

PATRICK E. McCLESKEY, MD, FAAD
Dermatologist, Department of Dermatology,
Kaiser Permanente, Oakland, California

TIEN VIET NGUYEN, MD
Bellevue Dermatology Clinic, Bellevue,
Washington

ANDREW J. PARK, MD
Department of Medicine, Kaiser Permanente
Oakland Medical Center, Oakland, California

Jon KLINT PEEBLES, MD
Department of Dermatology, Kaiser
Permanente Mid-Atlantic Permanente Medical
Group, Rockville, Maryland

DANIELLE J. POLIN, BA
Department of Dermatology, Stanford
University School of Medicine, Redwood City,
California

LAURA RAGMANAUSKAITE, BS
Department of Dermatology, Emory University
School of Medicine, Atlanta, Georgia

ANDREW V. RUOSS, MA, PhD
Dean of Teaching and Learning, The
Greenwich Country Day School, Greenwich,
Connecticut

KAVITA Y. SARIN, MD, PhD
Department of Dermatology, Stanford
University School of Medicine, Redwood City,
California

MARYANNE M. SENNA, MD
Department of Dermatology, Massachusetts
General Hospital, Harvard Medical School,
Boston, Massachusetts

RAHUL SETH, MD, FACS
Associate Professor, Facial Plastic and
Reconstructive Surgery, UCSF Department of
Otolaryngology–Head and Neck Surgery
(OHNS), San Francisco, California

WILLIAM R. SHORT, MD, MPH
Department of Medicine, Division of Infectious
Diseases, Perelman School of Medicine,
University of Pennsylvania, Philadelphia,
Pennsylvania

ALEXANDER SINCLAIR, MD
Director, Transgender Center, Southern
California Hospital System, Culver City,
California

JONATHAN M. SYKES, MD
Professor Emeritus, Facial Plastic Surgery, UC
Davis Medical Center, Sacramento, California,
Director, Facial Plastic Surgery, Roxbury
Institute, Beverly Hills, California

HOWA YEUNG, MD, MSc
Department of Dermatology, Emory
University School of Medicine, Atlanta,
Georgia

Contributors

WILLIAM R. SHORT, MD, MPH
Department of Medicine, Division of Infectious Diseases, Perelman School of Medicine, University of Pennsylvania, Philadelphia, Pennsylvania

ALEXANDER SINCLAIR, MD
Director, Transgender Center, Southern California Hospital System, Culver City, California

JONATHAN M. SYKES, MD
Professor Emeritus, Facial Plastic Surgery, UC Davis Medical Center, Sacramento, California; Director, Facial Plastic Surgery, Roxbury Institute, Beverly Hills, California

HOWA YEUNG, MD, MSc
Department of Dermatology, Emory University School of Medicine, Atlanta, Georgia

Contents

and those in the public and insurance policy sectors. These are not only professional deficiencies but also perpetuate discrimination, limit access to health care, and lead to poor health outcomes. Research supports the notion that acquiring skills and knowledge through dedicated training programs leads to more compassionate and competent care for LGBTQIA patients.

to prevent HIV infection. The most common PrEP regimen involves taking a single pill daily and is very effective in reducing risk of HIV infection, with few adverse effects. Barriers to PrEP access exist for MSM and transgender persons. Dermatologists can help combat the ongoing HIV epidemic among MSM, transgender persons, and others by understanding why, when, and how PrEP should be considered as an HIV prevention approach.

operations, emerging technologies and EHRs, clinic culture, clinic environment and resource availability, and provider and staff education are all characteristics of healthcare clinics that can be improved to better facilitate high-quality dermatologic care for LGBT patients.

Trainee Exposure and Education for Minimally Invasive Gender-Affirming Procedures   277

Brittany Buhalog, Jon Klint Peebles, Matthew Mansh, Esther A. Kim, Philip Daniel Knott, William Hoffman, Rahul Seth, Andre Alcon, and Sarah Tuttleton Arron

Minimally invasive gender-affirming procedures (MIGAPs), which aim to align gender identity and expression for transgender and gender-nonbinary patients in a way that is safe, effective, and semipermanent or reversible, are gaining in popularity. This article assesses the current amount of trainee exposure in clinic and didactic sessions in core procedural specialties nationwide via survey study of program directors. Low exposure of residents and fellows to MIGAPs was observed overall and a lack of procedure-specific education. In an effort to provide excellent patient care, promote cultural humility, and improve patients' quality of life, further education regarding these procedures is necessary.

Incorporating Lesbian, Gay, Bisexual, and Transgender Training into a Residency Program   285

Joseph W. Fakhoury and Steven Daveluy

Lesbian, gay, bisexual, and transgender (LGBT) patients experience vast health care disparities. Numerous government and professional organizations have attempted to address these disparities by calling for improvement in LGBT health and increased research endeavors. Despite these initiatives, residents still receive inadequate education and training in LGBT health. Here, the authors review these shortcomings and provide a framework for how to improve resident education and training in LGBT health. They describe methods of curricular enhancements and departmental/institutional climate optimization to improve resident competency. Finally, they discuss how LGBT-competent physicians can publicize their expertise and improve overall LGBT health care delivery.

DERMATOLOGIC CLINICS

SERIES OF RELATED INTEREST

Facial Plastic Surgery Clinics
Available at: http://www.facialplastic.theclinics.com/
Surgical Oncology Clinics
Available at: https://www.surgonc.theclinics.com/

THE CLINICS ARE AVAILABLE ONLINE!
Access your subscription at:
www.theclinics.com

Preface

A New Era of Care for the Lesbian, Gay, Bisexual, and Transgender Community

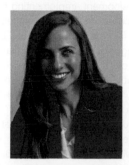 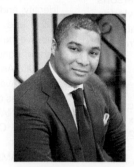

Lauren Meshkov Bonati, MD, FAAD   Jared Jagdeo, MD, FAAD

Editors

Lesbian, gay, bisexual, and transgender (LGBT) awareness in the United States is growing. As individuals from these unique communities take on increasingly visible and prominent roles in society, in politics, and in the mainstream media, the general public will look to leaders in medicine to set a precedent of Inclusion and nonprejudice.

LGBT care is an important timely topic in medicine. Health disparities within the LGBT patient population is a current focus of both the Healthy People 2020 initiative and the Association of American Medical Colleges, which recommends medical school curricula incorporate LGBT health competency.[1,2] High-impact journals and widely circulated new-blasts like *Medscape* regularly feature articles on LGBT issues and highlight the need for further education and competency in this space.[3-5]

While LGBT medicine is growing as a whole, dermatologic care for these patients remains understudied. This important gap was noted in the March 2018 *Journal of the American Medical Association* Dermatology research letter entitled, "Paucity of Lesbian, Gay, Bisexual, and Transgender Health Related Content in the Basic Dermatology Curriculum."[6] As the dermatologic community strives to learn how to best care for this population medically, there is also a need for better instruction on the delivery of aesthetic interventions. Data on the effectiveness of noninvasive cosmetic treatments for changing gender perception will enhance our ability to address gender dysphoria.

Despite growing awareness in the media and in medicine, there remains stigma, poor health care access, and lack of institutional policies and protections for LGBT patients. The LGBT community disproportionately suffers higher rates of substance abuse, mental health conditions, eating and body image disorders, obesity, early-onset disabilities, and sexually transmitted infections, including human immunodeficiency virus. They have lower rates of preventative cancer screenings and often rate themselves as having "poor health" more often than non-LGBT patients. These individuals are in desperate need of a safe space to address their medical and aesthetic concerns. We, as dermatologists, possess the knowledge and skills to help improve the lives of LGBT patients.

In this issue of *Dermatologic Clinics*, we address a wide range of LGBT topics, from the management of treatment-associated acne in LGBT persons to gender-specific relevant dermatoses, the

Dermatol Clin 38 (2020) xiii–xiv
https://doi.org/10.1016/j.det.2019.11.001

benefits of noninvasive cosmetic procedures, and how to make your clinical practice LGBT friendly. Other highlights include historical perspectives on LGBT care, testimonials from LGBT patients, and the status of current policy and insurance coverage for LGBT persons. We anticipate that this issue will serve as a useful resource for clinicians that provide skin care for LGBT persons and those looking to expand their knowledge base. It is our duty as leaders in dermatology and medicine as a whole to be on the forefront of change for the LGBT population.

Lauren Meshkov Bonati, MD, FAAD
Mountain Dermatology Specialists
PO Box 2819
Edwards, CO 81632, USA

Jared Jagdeo, MD, FAAD
SUNY Downstate Medical Center
Department of Dermatology
450 Clarkson Avenue
Box 46
Brooklyn, NY 11203, USA

E-mail addresses:
Lauren.bonati@gmail.com (L.M. Bonati)
jrjagdeo@gmail.com (J. Jagdeo)

REFERENCES

1. Office of Disease Prevention and Health Promotion. Lesbian, gay, bisexual, and transgender health. Healthy people. 2020. Available at: https://www.healthypeople.gov/2020/topics-objectives/topic/lesbian-gay-bisexual-and-transgender-health. Accessed March 30, 2018.
2. Advisory Committee on Sexual Orientation, Gender Identity, and Sex Development. Implementing curricular and institutional climate changes to improve health care for individuals who are LGBT, gender nonconforming, or born with DSD. Washington, DC: Association of American Medical Colleges; 2014. Available at: https://members-aamc-org.eresources.mssm.edu/eweb/upload/Executive%20LGBT%20FINAL.pdf. Accessed March 30, 2018.
3. Torke AM, Carnahan JL. Optimizing the clinical care of lesbian, gay, bisexual, and transgender older adults. JAMA Intern Med 2017;177(12):1715–6.
4. Transgender patients: tips for your practice. Medscape 2017.
5. Do ask. Do treat. Experts discuss cultural and medical competencies of caring for lesbian, gay, and bisexual patients. AAD 2017.
6. Park AJ, Katz K. Paucity of lesbian, gay, bisexual, and transgender health related content in the basic dermatology curriculum. JAMA Dermatol 2017.

Historical and Current State of Dermatologic Care for Sexual and Gender Minority Populations

Yi Chun Lai, MD, MPH[a], Maryia Kazlouskaya, BA[b],
Viktoryia Kazlouskaya, MD, PhD[a],*

KEYWORDS

- LGBTQ • Sexual and gender minority • Health disparity

KEY POINTS

- The lesbian, gay, bisexual, transgender, and queer or questioning/sexual and gender minority (LGBTQ/SGM) community has witnessed significant advances in equality and access to care over the past several decades.
- Dermatologists working in the contemporary environment should keep historical perspectives in mind and be cognizant of various aspects of providing care to the LGBTQ/SGM population.
- Dermatologists play an ever-increasing role In LGBTQ/SGM care, both medically and aesthetically.
- Active participation in professional organizations serving the LGBTQ/SGM population and implementation of education in undergraduate and graduate medical education are important ways to provide culturally competent care.

INTRODUCTION

The lesbian, gay, bisexual, transgender, and queer or questioning (LGBTQ)/sexual and gender minority (SGM) community makes up 2.7% to 5.3% of the U.S. population.[1,2] The community is growing partly because of decrease in bias and willingness to openly identify as LGBTQ/SGM.[2,3] As a result, there is an increasing demand in the medical care specifically oriented towards this group. Studies have shown that LGBTQ/SGM patients often experience barriers to healthcare due to prejudice, stigmatization, and lack of understanding for specific medical problems by physicians. Since the LGBTQ/SGM group is diverse and includes men who have sex with men (MSM), women who have sex with women (WSW), transgender individuals, and those who are unsure about their gender identity, education on how to provide medically appropriate and culturally sensitive care for these patients is essential.[4]

Dermatologists' role in the care of LGBTQ/SGM patients includes managing cutaneous manifestations of sexually transmitted infections (STIs), adverse effects of hormone replacement therapy, complications of gender-affirming surgery (GAS), and performing cosmetic procedures to enhance desirable physical characteristics.[5] This article aims to review the historical perspectives on the evolution of dermatologic care for LGBTQ/SGM population, discuss the establishment of various medical and dermatologic associations dedicated to their health, and define directions for future research and improvement.

a SUNY Downstate Medical Center, 450 Clarkson Avenue, Brooklyn, NY 11203, USA; b Queens College, CUNY, 65-30 Kissena Blvd, Flushing, NY 11367, USA
* Corresponding author.
E-mail address: viktoriakozlovskaya@yahoo.com

Dermatol Clin 38 (2020) 177–183
https://doi.org/10.1016/j.det.2019.10.001
0733-8635/20/Published by Elsevier Inc.

HISTORICAL PERSPECTIVE: PROFESSIONAL ORGANIZATIONS

Less than a century ago, homosexuality was regarded as an illness and remedies such as psychotherapy and castration have been proposed by some physicians to treat the condition.[6,7] Despite Alfred Kinsey's research in 1948, demonstrating that human sexuality is a continuum between pure homosexuality and heterosexuality, MSM and WSW continued to suffer from social rejection for decades.[6] In 1952, *homosexuality* was classified in the first edition of *Diagnostic and Statistical Manual of Mental Disorders* (DSM-I) as a "sociopathic personality disturbance."[7] One year later, President Eisenhower issued an executive order that prohibited lesbian and gay applicants from obtaining a federal job, leading to the popularization of conversion therapy, psychoanalysis, and even lobotomy.[8,9] Often, patients were coerced into undergoing therapies that have dire psychological consequences. It was not until 1973 that the diagnosis of homosexuality was removed from the DSM-II.[8] Finally, in 2015, the Obama administration banned the use of conversion therapy for minors, a legislation that has currently passed in only a few states (California, New Jersey, Oregon, Washington, D.C., and Illinois).[10]

In the early 1980s, dermatologists began to observe Kaposi sarcoma and oral candidiasis in MSM and were among the first to identify cutaneous manifestations of a newly recognized condition.[9] The constellation of findings was later defined by the Centers for Disease Control and Prevention (CDC) as acquired immunodeficiency syndrome (AIDS). Dermatologists have since diagnosed infectious and noninfectious dermatologic issues that are prevalent among the LGBTQ/SGM community and continue to be an integral part of medical care for these patients.

To address healthcare disparities faced by the LGBTQ/SGM community, various organizations were established to expand research efforts, provide funding, and formulate policy and recommendations. The Gay and Lesbian Dermatology Association (GALDA [www.glderm.org]) was among the first to raise awareness on LGBTQ/SGM health issues. GALDA aims to offer mentorship and professional advancement for dermatologists serving the community and provides a network to assist trainees without financial resources.[10] The group meets yearly at the American Academy of Dermatology (AAD) to exchange ideas, develop LGBTQ-related research, and discuss advocacy issues.

The GLMA: Health Professionals Advancing LGBTQ Equality, formed in 1981, is the largest medical organization for LGBTQ healthcare professionals (previously known as the Gay and Lesbian Medical Association [www.glma.org]). Originally established to address the human immunodeficiency virus (HIV)/AIDS epidemic, the GLMA agenda now includes cancer prevention, substance abuse, mental health, and access to care. GLMA also participates in various health care reforms, such as improving access and coverage for HIV patients under the Patient Protection and Affordable Care Act and promoting adoption of nondiscrimination and visitation policies for LGBTQ patients and families.[11] In 2007, the GLMA, in collaboration with the Human Rights Campaign Foundation, created the Healthcare Equality Index to evaluate an institution's LGBTQ-related policies and help facilities offer more equitable care for these patients. In addition, the GLMA promotes cultural competency education to help providers better address LGBTQ/SGM specific needs.[11] The GLMA also provides a list of LGBTQ-friendly providers, which include 63 dermatologists and 45 cosmetic medicine specialists.

An expert research group (ERG) on LGBTQ health was established in 2016 to provide educational resources for physicians. Numerous publications, continuing medical education articles, lectures, and grand rounds on LGBTQ/SGM health were among the ERG's various accomplishments.[12–16] It also helped develop the LGBTQ section for the AAD, created a transgender dermatology hands-on session at the 2019 AAD annual meeting, established dermatology representation in the newly formed LGBTQ Health Specialty Section Council at the American Medical Association, and drafted a comment on the Department of Veterans Affairs' proposed rule to exclude gender alterations from medical benefits package.

HISTORICAL PERSPECTIVE: TRANSGENDER DERMATOLOGY

Approximately 0.6% of the population in the U.S. identify themselves as transgender. *Transsexualism*, a term first coined in 1953 by Harry Benjamin, an American endocrinologist and champion of transgender people, illustrates an incongruity between sex assigned at birth and gender identity.[17] In 1980, transsexualism was classified in the DSM-III as a gender identity disorder. It was not until 2013 when the term, *gender identity disorder*, was replaced with *gender dysphoria* in DSM-V.[18] The U.S. Department of Health and Human Services recommended the inclusion of gender identity and sexual orientation data in electronic health records in 2015 to further facilitate the delivery of patient-centered care.[19]

The first GAS was performed in the early twentieth century. It took approximately a century of transgender activism for GAS to gain widespread acceptance in the medical community. Initially, the procedure was self-paid and performed in private institutions only. Finally, Medicare started providing coverage for GAS in 2014.[20] Surgical intervention, however, is only one aspect in the management of gender dysphoria, which usually requires a multidisciplinary team of specialists including dermatologists. In addition to surgeries, transgender patients often need lifelong hormone replacement therapy. The rise in these gender-affirming procedures makes dermatologists particularly essential in managing the cutaneous complications of these treatments.

Prior to the 1960s, there was no consensus on medical, surgical, or psychiatric evaluation for transgender patients. As a result, they suffered from unnecessary psychiatric therapies, incarceration, and discrimination. In response to this, the World Professional Association for Transgender Health (WPATH), formerly known as the Harry Benjamin International Gender Dysphoria Association, was formed in 1979. WPATH seeks to establish the highest standards of care for transsexual, transgender and gender nonconforming individuals all over the world (https://www.wpath.org). WPATH recently released the seventh edition of its *Standards of Care*, a manual that provides clinical guidance and evidence-based recommendations for transgender care, with the first version published in 1979.[21] The *International Journal of Transgenderism* is the official WPATH journal for current research on transgender health issues. WPATH also maintains an international registry of providers across multiple specialties that are involved in the care of transgender patients. Dermatologists, however, are underrepresented in WPATH, with only 1 provider currently listed in the U.S.

COMMON DERMATOLOGIC ISSUES IN LESBIAN, GAY, BISEXUAL, TRANSGENDER, AND QUEER OR QUESTIONING DERMATOLOGY
Human Immunodeficiency Virus/Sexually Transmitted Infections and Other Infectious Diseases

Heightened interest in LGBTQ/SGM care is reflected by a recent increase in the number of relevant publications. A considerable number of articles focus mainly on AIDS and other STI-related problems. This section reviews the current knowledge on common dermatologic issues in this population and discusses future direction for research and improvement.

As MSM are more likely to have STIs, HIV, viral hepatitides, methicillin-resistant *Staphylococcus aureus*, invasive meningococcal disease, and Kaposi sarcoma, a comprehensive sexual history should be elicited to guide appropriate screening and/or interventions.[12,13] **Table 1** summarizes the recommendations from the CDC and U.S. Preventive Services Task Force on HIV/STI screening, vaccination, and prophylaxis in MSM. Contrary to popular belief that WSW are a low-risk group for having HIV and STIs, they can acquire these infections from current and past male or female partners.[22] In addition, due to a lower perceived risk of STIs and no risk for pregnancy, WSW are less inclined to practice safe sex, obtain human papillomavirus (HPV) vaccination, and undergo Pap smear regularly.[12,13] The same recommendations for HIV/STI screening and vaccination for heterosexual women apply to sexual minority women.[12,13]

Recently, there has been a rise in the incidence of lymphogranuloma venereum among MSM in Europe, which usually causes anorectal and, rarely, urethral infections.[23] Although there is no current screening guideline for lymphogranuloma venereum, it may be warranted in cases of proctitis of unknown etiology.

Transgender Health

Dermatologists play a significant role in the care of transgender patients both before and after GAS. Complications of GAS are not uncommon and include difficulty urinating, unwanted hair growth, formation of hairballs, as well as vaginal discharge, shortening, and stenosis.[26,27] One recent meta-analysis showed that 32.5% of male-to-female transgender patients experienced GAS-related complications and 21.7% of them required re-operations.[26] Data have shown that transgender patients are less likely to have health insurance.[28] Moreover, not all insurance policies provide coverage for GAS, thus posing a financial barrier for transgender patients to achieve their desired physical transformation. Some patients have to cover costs out of pocket or even seek surgical care from less qualified providers outside of the U.S., further increasing the risk of complications and loss to follow-up.

Recent evidence suggests that the microflora of the neovagina is different from that of cisgender women and resembles either normal skin, intestinal, or bacterial vaginosis microflora.[25] This explains the high rates of vaginal irritation, discharge, and symptomatic candidiasis experienced by these patients.[29,30] There are also

Table 1
Recommendations from the Centers for Disease Control and Prevention and the US Preventive Services Task Force on human immunodeficiency infection/sexually transmitted infection screening, vaccination, and prophylaxis in men who have sex with other men

Infections	Screening	Vaccination/Prophylaxis	Comment
HIV[24,25]	Unknown or negative status, had or whose partner(s) had >1 sexual partner since last visit Screen annually; consider every 3–6 mo if high risk[a]	PrEP: emtricitabine-tenofovir disoproxil fumarate once daily nPEP: 28-d course of 3-drug antiretroviral regimen ≤72 h after a nonoccupational exposure	PrEP indication • Adult man • Negative HIV status • Any male sex partners in the past 6 mo • Not in a monogamous relationship with a recently tested, HIV-negative man AND at least 1 of the following • Any anal sex without condoms in the past 6 mo • A bacterial STI diagnosed or reported in the past 6 mo
Syphilis	Sexually active in the past year or since the last test; screen annually; consider every 3–6 mo if high risk[a]		
Gonorrhea and chlamydia	Screen annually at all 3 sites (pharynx, urethra, rectum); consider every 3–6 mo if high risk[a]		Nucleic acid amplification tests preferred at all anatomic sites
Hepatitis B	No previous vaccination, or previous/current infection; 1-time screening	2-dose or 3-dose series, depending on vaccine	
Hepatitis C	HIV-positive status; 1-time screening	3-dose series	
HPV		3 doses of 4-valent or 9-valent vaccine; 2 doses if 11–12 y of age	MSM should receive HPV vaccine through 26 y of age
Meningococcus		2-dose series of conjugated vaccine for serotypes A/C/W/Y	HIV-positive above 2 y of age

Abbreviations: nPEP, nonoccupational postexposure prophylaxis; PrEP, pre-exposure prophylaxis.
[a] If patient is receiving pre-exposure prophylaxis for HIV, or if patient and/or his partner(s) have multiple partners. Patient should receive HIV testing every 3 months as well as syphilis, gonorrhea, and chlamydia test at least every 6 months.

reports indicating that HPV-associated squamous cell carcinoma and lichen sclerosis may be more common among transgender women due to chronic inflammation from surgical procedures.[27,28] More research, however, is needed to further elucidate these relationships and help guide specific recommendations for screening.[31–33]

Transgender patients taking cross-sex hormone therapy may experience cutaneous adverse effects, such as acne vulgaris and androgenetic alopecia for transgender men and melasma for transgender women. Treatment of severe acne in transgender men often requires the use of isotretinoin. Those who are started on isotretinoin, a teratogen, must register with iPLEDGE as mandated by the U.S. Food and Drug Administration (FDA) in 2006. Currently, iPLEDGE classifies patients into only 3 groups, namely, males, females of reproductive potential, and females of nonreproductive potential. This raises an important issue on how to categorize transgender patients on iPLEDGE as it classifies patients based on assigned sex at birth, which may be unacceptable or even offensive to some individuals.[20,34] It has been advocated that iPLEDGE adopts a classification scheme based on pregnancy potential rather than sex/gender.[20,34] Dermatologists should also be cognizant of transgender patients' reproductive potential based on anatomy and discuss contraception and pregnancy testing accordingly.[30,31] The ERG on LGBTQ/SGM, together with iPLEDGE and the FDA, recently initiated the process of creating a gender-neutral electronic registering program.

Cosmetic Dermatology

Recently, there has been a growing demand for cosmetic procedures among LGBTQ/SGM patients. A cross-sectional study using an anonymous online survey showed that transgender patients did not rate genital surgery as a top priority.[35] Instead, they preferred procedures that visually enhance their gender-specific features. For instance, transgender men prioritized mastectomy, whereas transgender women preferred facial procedures, such as neuromodulators, fillers, and facial plastic surgery.[35] Laser hair removal remained the most commonly utilized procedure among both sexes, highlighting the importance of procedural dermatology in the transitioning process.[35]

Dermatologists are knowledgeable about differences in anatomic features of male and female faces and, therefore, play a central role in addressing the unique aesthetic needs of transgender patients.[36] HIV-associated facial lipoatrophy, which affects 10% to 80% of patients living with HIV worldwide, is a condition that historically and disproportionately affects LGBTQ/SGM patients. Fillers represent an effective treatment modality for this condition.[37] Currently, Sculptra (Galderma Laboratories, L.P., Switzerland Fort Worth, Texas) (poly-L-lactic acid) and Radiesse (Merz Pharmaceutical, Raleigh, NC) (calcium hydroxylapatite) are the only FDA-approved fillers for this indication, but a recent study has demonstrated the safety, efficacy, and versatility of hyaluronic acid fillers for treating HIV-associated facial lipoatrophy.[38]

For the LGBTQ/SGM community, cost remains an important barrier to obtain cosmetic procedures. Although GAS is covered by some insurances, including Medicare/Medicaid, facial and body contouring procedures are not and can be cost-prohibitive. The LGBTQ/SGM population is, as a result of limited access to health care, more likely to receive aesthetic treatments from unlicensed providers. This makes them more susceptible to undesirable consequences, such as the injection of foreign materials.[39] Serious complications, such as foreign-body granulomas, silicone migration or embolism, infections, ulceration, disfiguration, autoimmune autoinflammatory syndrome, and even death, have been reported.[40,41] Training dermatologists to provide LGBTQ/SGM specific cosmetic treatments, educating these patients to avoid receiving procedures from unqualified providers, and expanding coverage to include gender-affirming cosmetic services for eligible individuals are of paramount importance in this community.

LACK OF EDUCATION AND RESEARCH IN DERMATOLOGY

A fundamental way to improve dermatologic care for the LGBTQ/SGM community is to incorporate relevant topics in residency and fellowship curriculums. In 2014, the Association of American Medical Colleges advocated for medical student education on the health needs of LGBTQ/SGM population.[42] Despite this initiative, research has shown that LGBTQ/SGM health issues are lacking in the basic dermatology curriculum.[43] The ERG on LGBTQ/SGM is currently working with the AAD to add relevant questions to the American Board of Dermatology Certification Examination questions bank.

Funding for LGBTQ/SGM-related research is scarce, with only 26% of LGBTQ/SGM studies being financed and mostly through nongovernmental organizations.[3] GLDA and GLMA are two major nongovernmental organizations that fund

LGBTQ/SGM-related research. The GLMA established the Lesbian Health Fund in 1992 for projects addressing the health needs of lesbians and sexual minority women. Other sources of funding include grants from individual institutions and dermatologic societies. For instance, the Dermatology Foundation 2020 Research Awards Program provides financial support for LGBTQ/SGM-related projects. The AAD and Women's Dermatologic Society also fund research projects on relevant topics.

SUMMARY

In conclusion, some progress has been made to promote health care equality for the LGBTQ/SGM population, however, there is still room for improvement. Over the past few decades, the medical community has moved in the right direction, but there remains a lack of proper training in cultural competency and basic knowledge. Although there are collaborative organizations dedicated to serving this growing population, dermatologists must play an increasing role in both the medical and aesthetic aspects of LGBTQ/SGM care. By creating a welcoming environment, using nonjudgmental language, and demonstrating respect for diversity, dermatologists can and should provide LGBTQ/SMG-friendly services.

DISCLOSURE

No conflicts of interest or financial ties to disclose.

REFERENCES

1. Gates GJ. Vermont leads states in LGBT identification. State of the States Gallup Politics; 2017. Available at: https://news.gallup.com/poll/203513/vermont-leads-states-lgbt-identification.aspx.
2. Gates GJ. In U.S., more adults identifying as LGBT. State of the States Gallup Politics; 2017. Available at: https://news.gallup.com/poll/201731/lgbt-identification-rises.aspx.
3. Snyder JE. Trend analysis of medical publications about LGBT persons: 1950-2007. J homosexuality 2011;58(2):164–88.
4. Katz KA, Furnish TJ. Dermatology-related epidemiologic and clinical concerns of men who have sex with men, women who have sex with women, and transgender individuals. Arch Dermatol 2005;141(10):1303–10.
5. Charny JW, Kovarik CL. LGBT access to health care: a dermatologist's role in building a therapeutic relationship. Cutis 2017;99(4):228–9.
6. Kinsey AC. Sexual behavior in the human male. Philadelphia: W. B. Saunders Co.; 1948.
7. Diagnostic and statistical manual of mental disorders. Washington, DC: American Psychiatric Association; 1952.
8. O'Neal CM, Baker CM, Glenn CA, et al. Heath: a controversial figure in the history of deep brain stimulation. Neurosurg Focus 2017;43(3):E12.
9. Haldeman DC. The practice and ethics of sexual orientation conversion therapy. J Consult Clin Psychol 1994;62(2):221–7.
10. Drescher J, Schwartz A, Casoy F, et al. The growing regulation of conversion therapy. J Med Regul 2016;102(2):7–12.
11. Radice M, Manfredini S, Ziosi P, et al. Herbal extracts, lichens and biomolecules as natural photo-protection alternatives to synthetic UV filters. A systematic review. Fitoterapia 2016;114:144–62.
12. Yeung H, Luk KM, Chen SC, et al. Dermatologic care for lesbian, gay, bisexual, and transgender persons: Epidemiology, screening, and disease prevention. J Am Acad Dermatol 2019;80(3):591–602.
13. Yeung H, Luk KM, Chen SC, et al. Dermatologic care for lesbian, gay, bisexual, and transgender persons: terminology, demographics, health disparities, and approaches to care. J Am Acad Dermatol 2019;80(3):581–9.
14. Admassu N, Pimentel MA, Halley MC, et al. Motivations among sexual-minority men for starting and stopping indoor tanning. Br J Dermatol 2019;180(6):1529–30.
15. Dodds M, Arron ST, Linos E, et al. Characteristics and skin cancer risk behaviors of adult sunless tanners in the United States. JAMA Dermatol 2018;154(9):1066–71.
16. Mansh MD, Nguyen A, Katz KA. Improving dermatologic care for sexual and gender minority patients through routine sexual orientation and gender identity data collection. JAMA Dermatol 2019;155(2):145–6.
17. Benjamin H. Transvestitism and transexualism. Int J Sexol 1953;7:12–4.
18. Association AP. Diagnostic and statistical of mental disorders. 5th edition. Arlington (VA): American Psychiatric Publishing; 2013.
19. Medicare and Medicaid programs; electronic health record incentive program—stage 3 and modifications to meaningful use in 2015 through 2017. Department of Health and Human Services, Centers for Medicare and Medicaid Services. Available at: https://www.federalregister.gov/documents/2015/10/16/2015-25595/medicare-and-medicaid-programs-electronic-health-record-incentive-program-stage-3-and-modifications. Accessed February 18, 2019.
20. Katz KA. Transgender patients, isotretinoin, and US food and drug administration-mandated risk evaluation and mitigation strategies: a prescription for inclusion. JAMA Dermatol 2016;152(5):513–4.

21. Standards of care for the health of transsexual, transgender, and gender nonconforming people. The World Professional Association for Transgender Health. 2001. Available at: https://www.wpath.org/publications/soc. Accessed February 18, 2019.

22. Everett BG. Sexual orientation disparities in sexually transmitted infections: examining the intersection between sexual identity and sexual behavior. Arch Sex Behav 2013;42(2):225–36.

23. de Vrieze NHN, Versteeg B, Bruisten SM, et al. Low prevalence of urethral lymphogranuloma venereum infections among men who have sex with men: a prospective observational study, sexually transmitted infection clinic in Amsterdam, the Netherlands. Sex Transm Dis 2017;44(9):547–50.

24. Centers for Disease Control and Prevention. US public health service: preexposure prophylaxis for the prevention of HIV infection in the United Statesd2017 update: a clinical practice guideline. Available at: https://www.cdc.gov/hiv/pdf/risk/prep/cdc-hiv-prep-guidelines-2017.pdf. Accessed February 18, 2019.

25. Moyer VA. Screening for HIV: U.S. preventive services task force recommendation statement. Ann Intern Med 2013;159(1):51–60.

26. Dreher PC, Edwards D, Hager S, et al. Complications of the neovagina in male-to-female transgender surgery: a systematic review and meta-analysis with discussion of management. Clin Anat 2018;31(2):191–9.

27. Suchak T, Hussey J, Takhar M, et al. Postoperative trans women in sexual health clinics: managing common problems after vaginoplasty. J Fam Plann Reprod Health Care 2015;41(4):245–7.

28. Lane M, Ives GC, Sluiter EC, et al. Trends in gender-affirming surgery in insured patients in the United States. Plast Reconstr Surg Glob Open 2018;6(4):e1738.

29. Weyers S, Verstraelen H, Gerris J, et al. Microflora of the penile skin-lined neovagina of transsexual women. BMC Microbiol 2009;9:102.

30. de Haseth KB, Buncamper ME, Ozer M, et al. Symptomatic neovaginal candidiasis in transgender women after penile inversion vaginoplasty: a clinical case series of five consecutive patients. Transgend Health 2018;3(1):105–8.

31. Bollo J, Balla A, Rodriguez Luppi C, et al. HPV-related squamous cell carcinoma in a neovagina after male-to-female gender confirmation surgery. Int J STD AIDS 2018;29(3):306–8.

32. McMurray SL, Overholser E, Patel T. A transgender woman with anogenital lichen sclerosus. JAMA Dermatol 2017;153(12):1334–5.

33. Mundluru SN, Larson AR. Medical dermatologic conditions in transgender women. Int J Womens Dermatol 2018;4(4):212–5.

34. Mundluru SN, Safer JD, Larson AR. Unforeseen ethical challenges for isotretinoin treatment in transgender patients. Int J Womens Dermatol 2016;2(2):46–8.

35. Ginsberg BA, Calderon M, Seminara NM, et al. A potential role for the dermatologist in the physical transformation of transgender people: a survey of attitudes and practices within the transgender community. J Am Acad Dermatol 2016;74(2):303–8.

36. Dhingra N, Bonati LM, Wang EB, et al. Medical and aesthetic procedural dermatology recommendations for transgender patients undergoing transition. J Am Acad Dermatol 2019;80(6):1712–21.

37. Alves MD, Brites C, Sprinz E. HIV-associated lipodystrophy: a review from a Brazilian perspective. Ther Clin Risk Manag 2014;10:559–66.

38. Ho D, Jagdeo J. Safety and efficacy of a volumizing hyaluronic acid filler for treatment of HIV-associated facial lipoatrophy. JAMA Dermatol 2017;153(1):61–5.

39. Pinto TP, Teixeira FDB, Barros C, et al. Use of industrial liquid silicone to transform the body: prevalence and factors associated with its use among transvestites and transsexual women in Sao Paulo, Brazil. Cad Saude Publica 2017;33(7):e00113316 [in Portuguese].

40. Kazlouskaya V, Ugorji R, Heilman E, et al. Painful ulcers on the anterior thigh: challenge. Am J Dermatopathol 2019;41(4):e33.

41. Soriano A, Butnaru D, Shoenfeld Y. Long-term inflammatory conditions following silicone exposure: the expanding spectrum of the autoimmune/inflammatory syndrome induced by adjuvants (ASIA). Clin Exp Rheumatol 2014;32(2):151–4.

42. Hollenbach AD, Eckstrand KL, Dreger A. Implementing curricular and institutional climate changes to improve health care for individuals who are LGBT, gender nonconforming, or born with DSD. Washington, DC: Association of American Medical Colleges; 2014.

43. Park AJ, Katz KA. Paucity of lesbian, gay, bisexual, and transgender health-related content in the basic dermatology curriculum. JAMA Dermatol 2018;154(5):614–5.

Health Care Inequities of Sexual and Gender Minority Patients

Erica Arnold, BS[a,b], Nikhil Dhingra, MD[a,c],*

KEYWORDS

- LGBTQ • Queer • Health inequalities • Health care disparities • Minority care • Implicit bias
- Public health

KEY POINTS

- Although great advances have been made in serving the LGBTQ community, a great deal of work is left to be done to better serve the sexual and gender minority community.
- A long-standing history leading to distrust with the system will require time to heal and overcome, and recent strides, namely in the United States and Europe, to perform community-based outreach are a first step toward achieving this goal.
- Sexual and gender minority patients experience a broad range of discrimination that affects their healthcare outcomes, and significant work is needed in order to ensure more inclusive healthcare for members of this minority population.

INTRODUCTION

Sexual and gender minority (SGM) individuals include, but are not limited to, those who identify as lesbian, gay, bisexual, transgender, and queer (LGBTQ). Today this term has been expanded to enable greater inclusion with broader identities such as queer, genderqueer, genderfluid, gender nonconforming, and nonbinary. Expanding on the distinct definitions of each term is beyond the scope of this review. SGM individuals are considered a marginalized and at-risk population, facing significant health care inequities when compared with heterosexual and cisgendered (ie, "gender-conforming") populations. They are more likely than heterosexual and cisgendered individuals to experience discrimination, bias, and dissatisfaction with the medical system.[1–7] This article provides a broad overview of systemic health care inequalities confronting SGM patients.

THE LESBIAN, GAY, BISEXUAL, TRANSGENDER, AND QUEER POPULATION AND HEALTH CARE

The past 50 years of advancing LGBTQ rights is closely linked to health care. The industry long cemented and endorsed anti-gay stigma, sanctioning it as acceptable for the general populace by pathologizing queerness. The first 2 iterations of the Diagnosis and Statistical Manual (DSM) of the American Psychiatric Association attributed LGBTQ identity to mental illness and disorder. It was not until the 1973 rewrite of the DSM when homosexuality was eliminated as a disorder, and even today there are areas of ambiguity within the manual that continue to reinforce stigma.[8,9] Until this paradigm shifted, the LGBTQ population were largely treated with hostility by the health care community, which had embraced the then acceptable belief that deviation away from heterosexuality was a condition needing

a Spring Street Dermatology, 73 Spring Street, Suite 303, New York, NY 10012, USA; b University of Utah School of Medicine, Salt Lake City, UT, USA; c Department of Dermatology, Icahn School of Medicine at Mount Sinai, New York, NY, USA

* Corresponding author. Spring Street Dermatology, 73 Spring Street, Suite 303, New York, NY 10012.
E-mail address: drdhingra@navaderm.com

Dermatol Clin 38 (2020) 185–190
https://doi.org/10.1016/j.det.2019.10.002

curative correction. The stigmatization and pathologization of LGBTQ individuals has had a lasting impact on the trust of the LGBTQ with the health care community. Retrospectively, the dismantling of the original DSM framework may be one of the more critical junctures in advancement of LGBTQ health care rights. It was only in 1987 with the DSM-III when health care embraced a more contemporary view of homosexuality from the psychiatric, and medical, community.[8]

Coinciding with this was another vital moment of intersection of the health care and LGBTQ communities, the AIDS epidemic, which spurred some of the greatest advances in SGM-focused health care through social activism. As large numbers of predominantly gay men perished, a broad movement coalesced to demand scientific discovery, epidemiologic analysis, research grants, and health care outreach for those affected, the LGBTQ community. Some of the most critical building blocks of SGM-related health care emerged from this era, and this time also highlighted the critical impact on a marginal community at odds with and ostracized by the health care industry. The deleterious effects of anti-LGBTQ stigma in medicine and the value of social justice reform coincided in convincing an industry to value their responsibility to provide care despite difference, stigma, and bias.

BIAS, ITS ORIGINS, AND THE ESTABLISHMENT OF HEALTH CARE DISPARITIES

The origins of health care disparities for SGM patients are intimately linked to long-held discriminatory and prejudicial sociopolitical views that infiltrate many fields, including health care. Furthermore, it is well established that inequalities in health care are compounded when SGM patients are also members of an ethnic or racial minority. A critical study published more than 2 decades ago in 1994 by Shatz and O'Hanlan[10] noted that nearly 90% of physicians surveyed witnessed verbal disparagement against LGBTQ patients while 67% of those surveyed witnessed inferior treatment provided to SGM-identifying minority patients. Despite the broad social and political gains achieved by the SGM community in the past decade, a 2015 study by Burke and colleagues[11] noted 50% to 80% of medical students surveyed exhibiting some degree of bias against SGM populations, suggesting slow progress within the medical community. SGM populations have experienced a surge in social and political victories in select countries in recent years. This would incorrectly suggest that anti-LGBTQ bias

in health care is historical rather than ongoing. Burke and colleagues' study, whose subjects notably are younger and theoretically more socially progressive, suggest possible mitigation, but perpetuation, of anti-SGM bias.

It is important to consider the 2 distinct forms of bias that weigh equally in generating discrimination against SGM patients: implicit and explicit. Explicit bias is fairly straightforward, defined loosely as conscious preconceptions about an individual or group that can be intentionally directed verbally or physically at a group. Implicit bias is a more ambiguous concept, characterized by subconscious discriminatory sentiment that can often persist unbeknownst to the holder of such biases. A 1989 study by psychologist Patricia Devine[12,13] assessed explicit and implicit bias with respect to race. She noted 2 groups of individuals, regardless of disparate vocalized beliefs concerning racial equality (ie, explicit vs implicit), held similar subconscious stereotype belief systems.

The Implicit Association Test is a standardized model for assessing implicit bias; in 2015 Sabin and colleagues[14] used this modality to assess health care provider bias toward sexual minorities. They looked at a multitude of caregivers, including physicians, nurses, and mental health providers, noting a "strong implicit preference for straight people…among heterosexual providers." They conclude that such implicit bias could contribute to larger health care inequalities for sexual minorities. Although this may seem incongruent with the Hippocratic Oath when it comes to medical decision making, the reality is that studies have suggested implicit and explicit bias of all forms to affect the care received by minority patients.

EFFECTS OF HEALTH CARE INEQUITIES IN SEXUAL AND GENDER MINORITY POPULATIONS

Anti-SGM bias has significant consequences on the health and well-being of LGBTQ individuals. This is best demonstrated by the framework of the minority stress theory, or the physical and psychological effects of prejudice on stigmatized minorities. In their extensive 2013 review, Lick and colleagues[15] summarize the deleterious effects of minority stress on LGBT individuals. They first note the more straightforward effects of psychological harm induced by minority stress before delineating a variety of evidence suggestive of its effects on LGBTQ physical health. The discussion of prejudice-induced stress on physical well-being is extensive and beyond the scope of this review; however, the meta-analysis by Lick and colleagues[15] serves as an excellent launch point for those interested in better understanding the proposed pathogenesis of anti-LGBTQ bias and poorer health outcomes.

A factor that makes difficult the assessment of anti-LGBTQ bias on health care inequalities is that unlike other more well-delineated minority group definitions, the LGBTQ community is remarkably multifaceted. LGBTQ, a so-called umbrella or collective term, is used to reference an entire minority population, which unfortunately can minimize the more individual experiences of each of its members. Intersectionality, for those unfamiliar, is the interplay of multiple identities that collectively shapes an individual's experiences. Studies of health care impact on SGM populations are currently broad, rarely taking into account or stratifying by other defining characteristics. Beyond LGBTQ identity, many do not take into account other risk factors for health care disparities, such as age, gender, racial, ethnic, socioeconomic, or religious differences. Thus, looking through an intersectional lens at health care disparities for SGM will be of vital importance to understanding the risks facing this highly diverse group. One study, for instance, by English and colleagues[16] looked at black, Latino, and multiracial gay and black men and noted that racial discrimination compounded the effects of sexual orientation discrimination, leading to higher rates of mental health and substance abuse.

Barriers to care notwithstanding, survey-based studies of LGBTQ individuals demonstrate significant distrust with the medical community, leading to delays in seeking care, poorer outcomes, and higher rates of morbidity and mortality.[6] This is compounded by lack of access to preventive health care measures directed at SGM individuals. The causes of such disparities are multiple, ranging from the aforementioned biases, to lack of SGM-specific medical education, to the disconnect between the health care and SGM communities.[7]

With regard to medical decision making, formally teasing the effects of bias on a clinician's approach to patients is complicated. Most physicians subconsciously rely on algorithms and categorization in approaching a patient, and biases also contribute, often in the setting of risk stratification. Dovidio and Fiske[17] discuss stereotype content models utilizing stereotypical characteristics stratified by identity group (ie, racial, gender, or sexual minority), noting that health care providers, like nonproviders, are susceptible to espousing stereotypes about groups. Although no formal studies have been done to assess implicit bias, health care outcomes, and the SGM population, similar studies for racial minority patients note poorer outcomes. For instance, Green

and colleagues[18] noted pro-white implicit bias was associated with a higher likelihood of encouraging thrombolysis for acute coronary syndrome, based on a stereotype of black Americans being less cooperative. It is also well established that provider bias carries an inherently higher risk of minimization of patients' concerns, which can have deleterious effects. Biases, thus, can have a significant effect on clinical outcomes for minority patients when compared with the heteromajority.

The health care needs of SGM patients are varied and broad. Health care professionals uncomfortable with taking a detailed sexual history may miss signs of impending suicide for an LGBTQ youth, inadvertently dismiss a patient's same-sex partner during a consultation, or fail to screen properly for conditions that disproportionately affect SGM patients. For instance, the risk of cervical cancer is underestimated in lesbian women, and they thus undergo a lower rate of screenings.[19] A 2007 study by Brandenburg and colleagues[20] noted higher rates of breast cancer in homosexual than heterosexual women. In 2014, Peitzmeier and colleagues[21] noted that female-to-male transgender patients were significantly more likely to have inadequate or poor-quality Papanicolaou smears. Numerous similar disparity-highlighting case reports and case series can be found in the literature.

Although bias may explain part of the discrepancies, lack of data for risk stratification is another reason. Perhaps the biggest limitation to better understanding LGBTQ health care is the lack of large-scale and long-term formal studies focused on the community. Fundamentally, a vast majority of longitudinal studies assessing risk factors have not stratified cohorts by sexual orientation or gender identity. Here, progress is slowly being made. UCSF's PRIDE (Population Research in Identity and Disparities for Equality) study, launched in 2015, is a first-of-its-kind longitudinal cohort study designed to assess the health care needs of SGM patient populations. It was crafted in response to a 2011 study by the Institute of Medicine (IOM) and the NIH, which cites the dearth of data as the biggest limitation for LGBTQ health care.[22,23] This "data desert," the report found, was vast and lacked knowledge of social, medical, and psychological factors affecting the SGM community. The IOM laid out a framework for investigation with 4 tentpole goals: (1) the minority stress model, as already discussed; (2) the life course perspective, aimed at delineating the impact of various life milestones on LGBTQ individuals; (3) the intersectionality model (discussed later); and (4) assessing social ecology, or an SGM individual's support network.[23] A 2013 report from the NIH took the IOM's recommendations to establish goals of study for federally funded works to better grasp the many different facets of LGBTQ health care. In this report, the emphasis heavily rested on the importance of advancing targeted public health research to ultimately enhance our understanding of the concerns affecting SGM patients. This emphasizes the importance of studies such as UCSF's, which may generate a more methodical, evidence-based framework through which to view and overcome LGBTQ inequalities in health care.[24]

INEQUALITIES FOR LESBIAN, GAY, BISEXUAL, TRANSGENDER, AND QUEER PATIENTS IN DERMATOLOGY

Inequalities and biases exist for LGBTQ individuals across all areas of health care, including dermatology. For smaller specialties, in particular, the aforementioned limitations of LGBTQ-focused health care data and training are further amplified.[25,26] Transgender-focused training, in particular, suffers the most prominent exclusion during education and training.[26] These education gaps, particularly when combined with individual implicit biases, limit providers' abilities to elicit sexual histories and ascertain risk and care-focused challenges specific to SGM populations, ultimately resulting in substandard health care and likely poorer outcomes.[25]

A dermatology-specific concern for LGBTQ individuals, for instance, includes sexually transmitted conditions, particularly at bodily sites of sexual practice outside of what are thought of as "heteronormative sites" of sexual interaction. In general, men who engage in sex with men (MSM, or bisexual men) have been shown to have higher prevalence of sexually transmitted infections including human immunodeficiency virus (HIV), herpes simplex virus, syphilis, human papilloma virus (HPV), and hepatitis. Among the most studied and widely discussed, owing to its historical significance, is the rate of HIV among MSM populations. According to the Centers for Disease Control and Prevention (CDC), in 2016 of all HIV diagnoses in the United States, 67% were in MSM and bisexual men. Incidence of HPV, including high-risk serotype infection and HPV-induced dysplasias and cancers of the anal, oral, and penile surfaces, are also higher in MSM populations. In 2016, 81% of all males diagnosed with syphilis were MSM.[27] Finally, MSM are at an increased risk for hepatitis A and B infections caused by oral-anal intercourse, which may indirectly be detected by a

dermatologist, for instance, when starting biologic therapies for unrelated conditions such as psoriasis.[27–29] The CDC has outlined HIV and other sexually transmitted disease screening timelines for members of the LGBTQ population such as MSM and transgender patients, which differ from those for heterosexual men and women, and will be of relevance for clinical care by dermatologists.[30]

Women who have sex with women (WSW) and bisexual women are members of the LGBTQ community for whom less research has been conducted. Because of the perceived lower risk of sexually transmitted infections along with the risk of pregnancy being taken away, many WSW report lower rates of preventive and screening measures, as previously noted. Data here suggest distinct modes of infection transmission for queer women, however, highlighting the importance of collecting more data for risk stratification and training.

For transgender patients, dermatologists and plastic surgeons offer a unique ability to care for the medical and semicosmetic needs of this population. Beyond treatment of infectious diseases as determined by the trans individual's sexual preferences and gender of their preferred partner, the trans population carries additional medical needs, including diseases of the hair and skin as induced by hormonal therapies or as induced by their preoperative biological gender. For instance, female-to-male patients may experience male pattern alopecia and severe acne secondary to testosterone therapy. Acne, in turn, may require isotretinoin, which runs into the predefined gender-based concerns of pregnancy delineated in iPLEDGE, highlighting when dermatologists should be aware of the needs of trans patients.[27,31] Cosmetic treatments, including those undergone by nonlicensed providers in an attempt to feminize or masculinize a patient, may lead to untoward complications such as nodules, infections, and ulcers, which dermatologists, too, should be aware of.[32,33]

ADDRESSING HEALTH CARE INEQUALITIES OF AT-RISK SEXUAL AND GENDER MINORITY POPULATIONS

Addressing and overcoming health care inequalities facing the LGBTQ community falls outside the purview of this review and is discussed elsewhere in this issue. However, by briefly emphasizing areas of weakness that permit for such inequity to permeate throughout health care, some clear and addressable areas of enhancement can be considered. Certainly, large-scale data collection emphasizing longitudinal data and risk stratification will greatly enhance the public health awareness of the needs of the LGBTQ community, as demonstrated by the NIH and IOM reports. Another area of enhancement is the creation of cultural competency models directed at the LGBTQ community. A 2011 study noted only 5 hours of medical education were dedicated to LGBTQ-specific competencies.[34] Interestingly, a meta-review by Butler and colleagues[35] notes that LGBT-focused cultural competency in its current form is too ambiguous to be effective, suggesting that the absence of data may preclude effective training. Diversifying the health care provider population, too, has been shown to positively enhance LGBTQ acceptance among heterosexual providers, as several studies have demonstrated.[14,24,36–39]

Although great advances have been made in serving the LGBTQ community, a great deal of work is left to be done to better serve the SGM community. A long-standing history leading to distrust with the system will require time to heal and overcome, and recent strides, namely in the United States and Europe, to perform community-based outreach are a first step toward achieving this goal.

DISCLOSURE

The authors have nothing to disclose.

REFERENCES

1. Katz-Wise SL, Hyde JS. Victimization experiences of lesbian, gay, and bisexual individuals: a meta-analysis. J Sex Res 2012;49(2–3):142–67.
2. Krieger N, Sidney S. Prevalence and health implications of anti-gay discrimination: a study of black and white women and men in the CARDIA cohort. Coronary artery risk development in young adults. Int J Health Serv 1997;27(1):157–76.
3. Pennant M, Bayliss M, Meads C. Improving lesbian, gay and bisexual healthcare: a systematic review of qualitative literature from the UK. Diversity & Equality in Health and Care 2009;6:193–203.
4. Streed CG Jr, Harfouch O, Marvel F, et al. Cardiovascular disease among transgender adults receiving hormone therapy: a narrative review. Ann Intern Med 2017;167(4):256–67.
5. Utamsingh PD, Richman LS, Martin JL, et al. Heteronormativity and practitioner-patient interaction. Health Commun 2016;31(5):566–74.
6. Zeeman L, Sherriff N, Browne K, et al. A review of lesbian, gay, bisexual, trans and intersex (LGBTI) health and healthcare inequalities. Eur J Public Health 2019;29(5):974–80.
7. Martos AJ, Wilson PA, Meyer IH. Lesbian, gay, bisexual, and transgender (LGBT) health services in the United States: origins, evolution, and contemporary landscape. PLoS One 2017;12(7):e0180544.
8. Drescher J. Out of DSM: depathologizing homosexuality. Behav Sci (Basel) 2015;5(4):565–75.
9. Drescher J. Queer diagnoses revisited: the past and future of homosexuality and gender diagnoses in DSM and ICD. Int Rev Psychiatry 2015;27(5):386–95.
10. Schatz B, O'Hanlan K. Anti-gay discrimination in medicine: results of a national survey of lesbian, gay, and bisexual physicians. San Francisco (CA): Gay and Lesbian Medical Association; 1994.
11. Burke SE, Dovidio JF, Przedworski JM, et al. Do contact and empathy mitigate bias against gay and lesbian people among heterosexual first-year medical students? A report from the medical student CHANGE study. Acad Med 2015;90(5):645–51.
12. Devine PG, Forscher PS, Austin AJ, et al. Long-term reduction in implicit race bias: a prejudice habit-breaking intervention. J Exp Soc Psychol 2012;48(6):1267–78.
13. Devine PG. Stereotypes and prejudice: their automatic and controlled components. J Personal Social Psychol 1989;56(1):5–18.
14. Sabin JA, Riskind RG, Nosek BA. Health care providers' implicit and explicit attitudes toward lesbian women and gay men. Am J Public Health 2015;105(9):1831–41.
15. Lick DJ, Durso LE, Johnson KL. Minority stress and physical health among sexual minorities. Perspect Psychol Sci 2013;8(5):521–48.
16. English D, Rendina HJ, Parsons JT. The effects of intersecting stigma: a longitudinal examination of minority stress, mental health, and substance use among black, latino, and multiracial gay and bisexual men. Psychol Violence 2018;8(6):669–79.
17. Dovidio JF, Fiske ST. Under the radar: how unexamined biases in decision-making processes in clinical interactions can contribute to health care disparities. Am J Public Health 2012;102(5):945–52.
18. Green AR, Carney DR, Pallin DJ, et al. Implicit bias among physicians and its prediction of thrombolysis decisions for black and white patients. J Gen Intern Med 2007;22(9):1231–8.
19. Curmi C, Peters K, Salamonson Y. Lesbians' attitudes and practices of cervical cancer screening: a qualitative study. BMC Womens Health 2014;14:153.
20. Brandenburg DL, Matthews AK, Johnson TP, et al. Breast cancer risk and screening: a comparison of lesbian and heterosexual women. Women Health 2007;45(4):109–30.
21. Peitzmeier SM, Reisner SL, Harigopal P, et al. Female-to-male patients have high prevalence of

unsatisfactory Paps compared to non-transgender females: implications for cervical cancer screening. J Gen Intern Med 2014;29(5):778–84.

22. Madhusoodanan J. UCSF researchers launch landmark study of LGBTQ community health. 2015. Available at: https://www.ucsf.edu/news/2015/06/130631/ucsf-researchers-launch-landmark-study-lgbtq-community-health. Accessed March 22, 2019.

23. The health of lesbian, gay, bisexual, and transgender people: building a foundation for better understanding. Washington (DC): National Academies Press; 2011.

24. NIH LGBT Research Coordinating Committee. Consideration of the Institute of Medicine (IOM) report on the health of Lesbian, Gay, Bisexual, and Transgender (LGBT) individuals. Bethesda (MD): NIH; 2013.

25. Cooper MB, Chacko M, Christner J. Incorporating LGBT health in an undergraduate medical education curriculum through the construct of social determinants of health. MedEdPORTAL 2018;14:10781.

26. Dubin SN, Nolan IT, Streed CG Jr, et al. Transgender health care: improving medical students' and residents' training and awareness. Adv Med Educ Pract 2018;9:377–91.

27. Yeung H, Luk KM, Chen SC, et al. Dermatologic care for lesbian, gay, bisexual, and transgender persons: epidemiology, screening, and disease prevention. J Am Acad Dermatol 2019;80(3):591–602.

28. Martin TCS, Rauch A, Salazar-Vizcaya L, et al. Understanding and addressing hepatitis C virus reinfection among men who have sex with men. Infect Dis Clin North Am 2018;32(2):395–405.

29. Shover CL, DeVost MA, Beymer MR, et al. Using sexual orientation and gender identity to monitor disparities in HIV, sexually transmitted infections, and viral hepatitis. Am J Public Health 2018;108(S4):S277–83.

30. CBC lesbian, gay, bisexual, and transgender health. Available at: https://www.cdc.gov/lgbthealth/index.htm. Accessed March 22, 2019.

31. Mundluru SN, Safer JD, Larson AR. Unforeseen ethical challenges for isotretinoin treatment in transgender patients. Int J Womens Dermatol 2016;2(2):46–8.

32. Dhingra N, Bonati LM, Wang EB, et al. Medical and aesthetic procedural dermatology recommendations for transgender patients undergoing transition. J Am Acad Dermatol 2019;80(6):1712–21.

33. Mundluru SN, Larson AR. Medical dermatologic conditions in transgender women. Int J Womens Dermatol 2018;4(4):212–5.

34. Obedin-Maliver J, Goldsmith ES, Stewart L, et al. Lesbian, gay, bisexual, and transgender-related content in undergraduate medical education. JAMA 2011;306(9):971–7.

35. Butler M, McCreedy E, Schwer N, et al. Improving cultural competence to reduce health disparities. Rockville (MD): Agency for Healthcare Research and Quality; 2016.

36. Cochran BN, Peavy KM, Cauce AM. Substance abuse treatment providers' explicit and implicit attitudes regarding sexual minorities. J Homosex 2007;53(3):181–207.

37. Cochran BN, Peavy KM, Santa AF. Differentiating LGBT individuals in substance abuse treatment: analyses based on sexuality and drug preference. J LGBT Health Res 2007;3(2):63–75.

38. Phelan SM, Burke SE, Hardeman RR, et al. Medical school factors associated with changes in implicit and explicit bias against gay and lesbian people among 3492 graduating medical students. J Gen Intern Med 2017;32(11):1193–201.

39. Malebranche DJ, Peterson JL, Fullilove RE, et al. Race and sexual identity: perceptions about medical culture and healthcare among Black men who have sex with men. J Natl Med Assoc 2004;96(1):97–107.

The Patient's Perspective
Reorienting Dermatologic Care for Lesbian, Gay, Bisexual, Transgender, and Queer/Questioning Patients

Andrew V. Ruoss, MA, PhD[a], William R. Short, MD, MPH[b], Carrie L. Kovarik, MD[c],*

KEYWORDS

- LGBTQ • Cultural competency • Cultural humility • Dermatology • Patients • Bias • Diversity

KEY POINTS

- The past decade has seen significant advancements in the care of lesbian, gay, bisexual, transgender, and queer/questioning (LGBTQ) patients, but these efforts have primarily taken the form of institutional policy changes and medical staff training in cultural competency rather than addressing individual perceived bias and personal awareness.
- As practitioners gain an awareness of their own biases and the many facets of their own personal identity, cultural humility encourages them to recognize each LGBTQ patient as the expert of that patient's intersectional identity.
- Overall, patients want to feel welcome with a greeting when a dermatologist comes in the room; questions regarding the patient history should not be forced or awkward but necessary and nonjudgmental; the physical examination should be done as it would be for any other patient (including a full genital/anal examination if needed); and any partner or family member should be included in health care discussions and decisions per the patient.

INTRODUCTION

As a social scientist, an architect for LGBTQ programs in education, and a patient, I was inspired to lead the authorship of this article, collaborating with medical practitioners in an effort to introduce new perspectives to patient care.

—Andrew V. Ruoss, PhD

As a physician with a diverse dermatology practice, it is important for me to learn about each of my patients with unbiased thoughtful concern. My clinic is a place where the patients should feel comfortable discussing their

sensitive dermatologic issues with no judgement. Instead of writing about my experience, I thought it was important for dermatologists to hear directly from LGBTQ patients.

—Carrie L. Kovarik, MD

The past decade has seen significant advancements in the care and representation of LGBTQ patients in American health care. These efforts have primarily taken the form of institutional policy changes and medical staff training in cultural competency—both with the aim of fostering more inclusive clinical environments. These developments highlight what is already known to be true: all physicians, including dermatologists, see

[a] The Greenwich Country Day School, Greenwich, CT 06830, USA; [b] Department of Medicine, Division of Infectious Diseases, Perelman School of Medicine, University of Pennsylvania, 3400 Spruce Street, Philadelphia, PA 19104, USA; [c] Department of Dermatology, Perelman School of Medicine, University of Pennsylvania, 2 Maloney Building, 3600 Spruce Street, Philadelphia, PA 19104, USA
* Corresponding author.
E-mail address: carrie.kovarik@pennmedicine.upenn.edu

Dermatol Clin 38 (2020) 191–199
https://doi.org/10.1016/j.det.2019.10.003
0733-8635/20/© 2019 Elsevier Inc. All rights reserved.

LGBTQ patients and need to be effective care providers. Perceived bias on the part of a health care provider can have dire consequences for the health of LGBTQ-identifying individuals, causing patients to withhold critical information and to avoid seeking treatment of potentially life-threatening conditions.[1] The efficacy of staff training and policy changes, however, is difficult to assess. Drawing from patient interviews and author expertise, this article discusses the patient experience as the starting point for the development of effective, inclusive policy. Looking to the related field of LGBTQ youth wellness and education and focusing on an integrative approach to LGBTQ health care within the University of Pennsylvania Health System,[2] the authors seek to reframe the discussion about the care of LGBTQ-identifying patients in dermatologic practices.

BEYOND MEDICINE: CULTURAL COMPETENCE AND CULTURAL HUMILITY

The significant advancements in LGBTQ health care have evolved within the broader reform of bias against all underrepresented patient populations.[3] Implementing antidiscrimination policies, staff bias training, and diversified hiring processes has allowed physician practices and health systems across the country to incorporate LGBTQ identities into their efforts and to better serve patients representing a wider range of racial, religious, and socioeconomic backgrounds.[4] Implicit bias — a provider's bias, frequently subconscious in its nature, against a particular personal identity[5] — has become the primary target of institutional education campaigns.[3] Cultural competence — training designed with the goal of the practitioner developing knowledge and understanding of cultural perspectives different from their own[6] — has emerged as the primary goal of these campaigns and has become best practice across medical fields. When limited to discrete, or annual, informational trainings, however, these efforts do not consistently engender an improved patient experience. A recent review of the efficacy of professional trainings on transgender identity suggests that the traditional model of one-off, outside consultant presentations can cause more harm than good (Green ER. 2014. Does Teaching Transgender Content Effectively Reduce Anti-Transgender Prejudice? The Assessment Findings from a National Study. Widener University, Chester, PA). Although there is evidence that shows that basic trainings should be considered an imperative part of an educational initiative to reduce bias and prejudice against transgender populations, they should be 1 component of a larger-scale, intentional program.

These data indicate that educative cultural competence approaches need to be supplemented with practical and consistent strategies for inclusive patient engagement.

Other professional fields that have undertaken similar changes in their treatment of LGBTQ individuals also can be looked to. From the field of law, for example, has emerged the concept of intersectionality, that examines an individual's experience under the law through the intersections of the many facets of that person's identity, including race, class, gender, and sexual identity.[7] The goal of cultural competence might push dermatologists to recognize their own biases related to race or to study the perspective of a gay or lesbian patient. Human identity, however, is known to be complicated, LGBTQ or otherwise. Dermatologic care can directly involve all facets of a person's public and private identity. Patients bring the privileges and anxieties — defined by the perspective of their racial, socioeconomic, gender, and sexual identities in broader society — into the examination room. Supplementing competence with the ability to engage with the complicated intersections of human identity could dramatically improve the quality of care provided by a dermatologist.

The field of education also shares medical practitioners' motivation to develop more effective best practices for supporting and empowering LGBTQ-identifying individuals. It is known that in both fields, ineffective communication can have serious consequences. Although potentially life-saving, health care can be hampered by a biased provider; the alienation of LGBTQ youth has produced a suicide rate approximately 3 times higher than that of their peers.[8] In response to these alarming statistics, schools, advocacy groups, and state and federal agencies have developed robust best practices for the care and education of LGBTQ youth.[9] One of the nation's leading LGBTQ wellness centers and education consultancies is the Mazzoni Center in Philadelphia, Pennsylvania. Elizabeth C. Kahn, who leads the center's education division, notes that her field's best practice has shifted beyond cultural competence to a far more expansive and intrinsic approach: "As a department, we have moved away from calling what we offer LGBTQ Cultural Competence trainings to inviting every organization to invest in an ongoing educational partnership with Mazzoni Center. Our goal is to initiate fundamental and sustainable organization culture change which increases inclusivity, visibility, safety, and recognition of LGBTQ community members." Kahn and her staff encourage organizations "to look beyond the 101 training" and to "recognize the significance of assessing multiple components of an organization's process and structure" as part of a long-term evolution.

Because gender and sexual identity applies to everyone, the most effective support of LGBTQ patients depends on a practitioner's own interrogation of personal identity.[10] Durable goals of institutional change rely on (1) leadership's clear communication of expectations to staff members and (2) creating an educational process free from judgment and focused on each employee's long-term personal development and education. To scaffold this process, Kahn describes how the Mazzoni Center has developed a reflective approach, designed to reach all stakeholders in an institution. In working with a massive organization with thousands of employees or a local medical practice with a handful of staff, the Mazzoni Center best practice centers on 5 core principles:

1. A top-down commitment is vital for any lasting organizational change.
2. Personal awareness and a willingness to self-assess, self-monitor, and grow are essential from each member of the organization.
3. Expectations for interpersonal behavior must be set by the organization to reinforce change and to hold all people accountable for their actions.
4. The voices of the most marginalized in the LGBTQ communities, like trans people of color, should be centralized.
5. Every effort should be made to continually reinforce the commitment to diversity and inclusive practices. For example, in hiring and promotion processes, in structural changes (accessible, gender-neutral bathrooms), in antidiscrimination policies, in protocol for disclosing harassment, and so forth.

The Mazzoni Center experience demonstrates that, in order to sustain any organizational change, it also is essential to establish internal advocates and change-makers. These individuals can continue to assess, reinforce, and update the improvements made from within the organization. According to Kahn, "this process starts by amplifying LGBTQ voices, specifically those of color, in all aspects of change and growth. We deeply believe that changes made to include and uplift the LGBTQ communities should come from the LGBTQ communities themselves." A core goal of institutional change for a dermatologic practice would thus be to recognize and amplify their LGBTQ stakeholders in a respectful and meaningful way, while maintaining appropriate trauma-informed boundaries.

A similar framing of self-reflective approaches to the intersections of identity has entered health care through the concept of cultural humility training. Beyond the goal of competency, this approach introduces the self-reflective element prioritized within education. Rather than the study of different identities, cultural humility techniques promote continual engagement in self-reflection and self-critique as lifelong learners and reflective practitioners.[11] In this way, the human resources of a medical practice become the clinical environment's greatest tool for effective engagement with patients. The goal in this approach is effective communication, not knowledge acquisition. As practitioners gain an awareness of their own biases and the many facets of their own personal identity, cultural humility encourages them to recognize each LGBTQ patient as the expert of that patient's intersectional identity.[12] This approach thus prioritizes the role of the patient as a partner in their own health care, rather than requiring the practitioner to become the expert on an identity. Perhaps reflective of the consistent interpersonal contact with patients at the core of the nurse's role, nursing schools have aggressively promoted the concept of cultural humility in their professional training.[13]

PATIENT PERSPECTIVES

Bringing together these concepts from education, law, and health care approaches can begin to be assembled for more effective engagement with LGBTQ patients. This article, however, moves beyond the conceptual discussion to understand concrete examples of practitioner engagement in the dermatology clinic. From a patient point of view, what does a culturally competent, reflective practitioner look like? How does the LGBTQ patient understand the intersections of their own identities? How do patients interpret the physical, verbal, and social cues of the practitioner?

Four different patient profiles are assembled, providing reflections on their experiences in clinical dermatology settings. The patients offer reflections that vary in their length, historical depth, and detail. By no means are these 4 individual perspectives—a white gay man; a black trans woman, a black gay man, and a white lesbian woman—sought to be representative as indicative of LGBTQ experience generally. The label LGBTQ, itself, is an increasingly insufficient acronym to encapsulate a wide range of identities.[14] Instead, the aim is to highlight clinical experiences from the patient perspective as a starting point from which to improve the LGBTQ patient experience in dermatologic practices. All patient names have been anonymized.

Patient 1 identifies as a gay, African American, cisgender man, age 52. Growing up in a low-income household in Reading, Pennsylvania, the patient keenly perceived the limiting factors that society placed on his identity, particularly pertaining to his race, sexuality, and socioeconomic status. He was "in the closet for a while" after childhood, and he knew of no physicians "like him" in Reading. When the patient sought treatment of human immunodeficiency virus (HIV) and human papillomavirus (HPV), he frequently withheld his sexual identity as well as his addiction to recreational drugs, from his physicians. After a few visits, he gained enough comfort with a dermatologist to disclose his sexual identity, and the dermatologist said that he would not see Patient 1 again "because he lied to him." When he moved to Philadelphia, the patient encountered providers who would make disparaging and dismissive remarks about his struggle with drug use or evinced discomfort related to his HIV status. In his professional and personal life, the patient felt the same anxieties that defined his medical care, where he could be denied employment and insurance for his sexual identity and HIV status.

Reflecting on his experience in the University of Pennsylvania LGBTQ Health Program, Patient 1 noted several approaches that his dermatologist and her medical staff took, which changed his experience of dermatologic care. First, his practitioner always shook his hand on entering and exiting the examination room. Dermatologic conditions, such as HPV, frequently generate discomfort and embarrassment within patients.[15] The simple, personal contact of the handshake eliminated many fears of physical judgment or perceptions of disgust in the provider-patient relationship. The patient noted that his provider was also "persistent" in her questioning, but she did not rush his disclosure of details. One may not share everything "on the first date," so to speak, and there was a tacit acknowledgment that it takes time to build a rapport. In this dermatologist's questioning—including body language, phrasing, and responses—Patient 1 noted, "there was no judgment, only concern," particularly related to sexual history. Her willingness to speak with other physicians "to get more ideas about his conditions" telegraphed a humility, which, combined with her clinical approach, conveyed that the provider was open to engagement with all potential facets of the patient's identity.

Patient 2 identifies as a white, lesbian, cisgender woman, age 74. The patient has perceived a range of physician biases and assumptions related to her intersectional identity, which have impeded her care. She reports that comments and questions from several clinical practitioners have suggested that she does not fit the "stereotype" for a gay woman. When she has told physicians that she has a "partner," she has "caught them off guard." In this way, her sexual identity also intersects with her gender identity, her physical appearance, and her age profile. She thinks that practitioners likely assume she is a heterosexual grandmother, and this prejudgement leads to a loss of rapport once they realize that she is gay. After cardiac surgery, for example, she consulted a plastic surgeon for reparative surgery. On the day of the procedure, Patient 2 brought her partner with her. The patient was asked to have her partner wait outside during preoperative care. Patient 2 recalls saying, "No, this is my partner." A member of the health care team said, "Partner?" After that, the conversation turned very cold and awkward. This was particularly jarring, given the anxiety and emotions that define the preoperative setting. It is in preoperative care that a patient can already feel the most powerless and "at the hands" of a physician. This only heightens a patient's awareness of any bias or judgment from the provider, related to the patient's identity. It is during the preparations for treatment or surgical procedure that the dermatologist and team should be most attuned to the perspective and well-being of the patient.

Importantly, this patient's experience also demonstrates how the physician's concept of identity also must extend beyond the individual patient, themselves. Partners, friends, and family members who identify as LGBTQ can represent critical elements of a patient's identity. Any perceived judgment or lack of openness related to these individuals can dramatically affect the physician-patient relationship and hamper quality of care. For example, it is of particular importance to Patient 2 that her practitioners acknowledge an important role for her partner in decision making and updates. Patient 2 reports that if she sees a new physician who responds in an awkward way to the introduction of a "partner," she often makes the effort to seek out a different physician in the practice. Although Patient 2 has been able to seek out and find many health care providers who do not respond to her sexual identity and gender in ways that "create barriers to her health and dermatology care," this also demonstrates how perceived bias on the part of the provider transfers to the patient the burden of seeking out and ensuring quality of care.

Patient 3 identifies as an African American, transgender woman, age 41. She is HIV positive and seeks concurrent care for her physical transition process and her HIV management. Describing her experiences of different medical practices, Patient 3 highlighted the importance of training for all employees within a clinical setting. "Just walking into a clinic," she began, "I immediately get looks from the front desk staff and I can see them whispering to each other." Although she attributes this to her appearance, the patient also spoke about the importance of pronoun use and name recognition for transgender patients. She is constantly misgendered, and providers "never" ask her for her preferred name. Instead, "they see that I look like a woman and yet they call me by the name I was given at birth." Once in the examination room, the patient feels that providers frequently cannot get past their bias and clearly convey a lack of understanding of transgender identity: "I try to find a clinic where they are comfortable with transgender individuals, but it is hard." This can present as a refusal of care, as the patient referenced dermatologists who were uncomfortable with injections for facial feminizations. Additionally, providers also may prematurely cut off essential questioning: "Not many doctors ask me about my sexual history and I am not sure why because I thought it was important [to my care]." In agreement with the other patients in this study, Patient 3 reports that she feels that this pattern puts the onus on the patient to seek out welcoming, informed providers—a process which can prove arduous and fatiguing: "when I get tired of this, I just stop seeking care for a while—It is very frustrating."

Only recently has the field of dermatology begun to develop best practices for the critical role that the dermatologist can play in the physical transformation and care of transgender patients.[16] Reflecting on her experiences, Patient 3 is in agreement with the other patients in this study, focusing on the importance of humility and openness to intersectional identities: "I think the most important thing is to connect with me as a patient. Do not assume anything. Ask me what name I preferred to be called. Do not be embarrassed to ask what type(s) of surgery I have had." Patient 3 urged that the basis for her most successful physician-patient relationships has been mutual respect. A key demonstration of this successful engagement is clear questioning. Patient 3 conveyed that any reticence to question the patient related to surgeries or therapies involved in physical transition can telegraph bias. "Ask me and I will tell you," the patient stated, "If you do not ask, I assume you do not…understand what types of surgeries can be done." Engaged questioning empowers the patient to enter into a collaborative relationship with the provider. Similarly, Patient 3 spoke to the importance of physical communication of openness and comfort, highlighted also by Patient 1 and Patient 4. Just as the handshake was critical to patients seeking

treatment of HPV, Patient 3 states that she was "fine with having a total body exam or genital exam." Because her primary goal was to seek out the best care, it was the demonstration of discomfort on the part of the provider that inhibited effective dermatologic care: "I think providers are more uncomfortable and it shows on their face [they are]."

Patient 4 identifies as a gay, white, cisgender man, age 30. He grew up in an affluent suburban household and is a highly educated professional. Although the facets of his identity represent a great deal of societal privilege, his case highlights unique dynamics of American dermatologic practice, particularly related to sexual identity. Despite his comparatively unencumbered access to high-quality health care, Patient 4 reported negative clinical experiences similar to those of Patient 1. For his initial treatments for HPV, Patient 4 sought care in 2 highly regarded suburban dermatologic practices, which, like many such practices, focus primarily on cosmetic procedures and on the treatment of skin cancer. In both practices, Patient 4 encountered dermatologists and nurses who exhibited clear discomfort with his condition. His first provider responded to the patient's disclosure of his reason for seeking treatment (HPV) by assuming "that he was gay, as they tend to see that with gay men." She then asked the patient "whether his parents and family knew about his lifestyle." Throughout treatment, the provider would not touch the patient, and "was distinctly uncomfortable—stuttering and looking away from him—when asking about sexual history." His next dermatologist "would not touch him, and had him examine himself" in lieu of any physical contact with the patient. This second provider then told Patient 4 "that, since HPV was incurable, he would never again be able to have an intimate relationship with someone."

Although many facets of Patient 4's identity would have otherwise made him feel welcome in these 2 dermatologic practices, he nonetheless found that his identity as a gay man inspired clear discomfort in his providers. Reflecting on his experience in the LGBTQ Health Program at the University of Pennsylvania, he echoed the importance of his dermatologist's "handshake," particularly related to his HPV diagnosis. He had taken to heart his previous provider's dismal assessment of his potential for future intimacy, which compounded his disgust with the physical appearance of warts. His new provider's calm questioning style "demonstrated no discernible reaction to his sexuality, or to any element of his story or concerns." This dermatologist was "clearly just interested in my wellbeing," Patient 4 stated, and all of her questions were "designed to get relevant information for my care." Recognizing the patient's anxiety, the provider "made sure to let me know that this was an extremely common issue" and also frequently injected humanizing questions and stories, which "lowered my anxiety and gradually built a social rapport between us." Patient 4's experience demonstrates the clear need for consistent cultural competence and humility training as well as training in a wider range of sexually transmitted infection–related care, even in well-resourced dermatologic practices.

TOWARD AN INCLUSIVE DERMATOLOGY PRACTICE

When examined together, these patient testimonies help reframe the perspective on the experience of LGBTQ patients in dermatology clinics. None of these patients expected the practitioners to be experts on LGBTQ identity. Even their positive clinical experiences did not require that. Rather, productive patient-dermatologist engagement occurred when the practitioner displayed humility, openness, and a lack of any prejudgment related to facets of a patient's identity. Consistent

practices like "the handshake" also added a physical connection that, although it may not be welcomed by all patients (and it is important to recognize that, as well), clearly indicates a genuine interest in building a relationship with the patient.

Pursuant to the goals for the provider and practice that the authors have put together (**Box 1**), several hospital systems have moved beyond a reliance on external consultants and trainings to introducing robust initiatives designed to construct internal networks of expertise in the care of LGBTQ patients.[17] Responding to motivations similar to those highlighted by the Mazzoni Center in the field of professional education, programs like the UCLA LGBTQ Health initiative, the New York-Presbyterian/Weill Cornell LGBTQ Task Force, the Cleveland Clinic LGBTQ health program, and the University of Pennsylvania LGBTQ Health Program, publicly identify health care providers experienced in the care of LGBTQ patients. Gathering these providers across the full range of specialties, such programs serve critical internal and external purposes. Internally, the program provides a network of expertise within the institution, on which other providers can draw for knowledge, guidance, and advice. Such

---

Box 1
Goals for the provider and for the practice

Approach: approach every case as a clean slate, and consciously focus on not making assumptions based on a patient's appearance, perceived age, or racial, gender, sexual, or socioeconomic identity. Continue this openness beyond the first meeting, understanding that trust and rapport are built over time, and crucial information may come from the patient only at a later time of their choosing.

Engagement: engage in honest self-reflection related to personal biases, fears, and discomforts. If uncomfortable when caring for LGBTQ-identifying people, then a plan should be made until these patients can be better served.

Staff and providers: if diversity, equity, and inclusion are goals of a practice, then those goals need to be telegraphed clearly to employees, patients, and potential patients. For staff, comprehensive, recurring, and consistent training related to cultural competence and cultural humility should be a clear investment of a practice. The practice also should work to recruit providers who demonstrate interest and strength in these fields. In application materials, these priorities should be highlighted. Questions that inspire self-reflection and probe an applicant's interest in equity and inclusion should be incorporated into interview processes.

Consistency: consistent training allows a dermatology practice to portray these goals as a process rather than a mandate. There is no one who can shift long-held perspectives or recognize their own biases after a single hour-long training. Medical practitioners should feel comfortable being honest and acknowledging biases from which they can work toward a more inclusive practice of medicine. The department or practice should structure ongoing conversations, instruction, observation, and feedback. No provider will ever be the expert on identity and always will have more to learn. This is particularly important in academic settings with residency programs and medical students.

Practice: policies matter only when they are practiced. Something as simple as a handshake completely shifted the experience of multiple patients within the University of Pennsylvania DERMATOLOGY DEPARTMENT. Create a regular, intentional opportunity within your practice for providers to share, without judgment, encounters that went well and those that did not. Reflect, as a team, on shared goals related to achieving the best possible outcome for all patients' experiences, including LGBTQ patients.

Box 2
Guidelines for effective questioning

General

- Legal name, name I prefer to be called (if different)
- Preferred pronoun?
- Gender (man, woman, trans [man to woman, woman to man], other)
- Sexual orientation (LGBTQ, other)
- Relationship status, living situation, children
- Profession/job/career
- Hobbies

Sexual history (if relevant)

- Are your sexual partners men, women, or both?
- Have you been tested for HIV?
- Determine sexually transmitted disease risk factors if relevant.

Gender, sexuality, and health care access

- Describe whether sexual/gender identity has been a barrier to health care? Why?
- Has your sexual/gender identity prevented you from getting care for a skin problem? For a skin problem that may have involved giving a sexual history or an examination of the genitals (if so, please give examples)?

Personal clinical experience

- Do you feel that you get the health care that you need?
- What has been the most difficult thing for you when accessing health care? dermatologic care specifically?
- Are there differences between your experiences with dermatology providers and providers in other medical specialties, or with general practitioners?

Personal perceptions of bias

- Have you ever felt discriminated against in a health care setting? Misunderstood?
- What were the results of you feeling that way?
- Has there been a difference in the way you feel when going to see a dermatologist specifically? When you see a dermatologist or doctor for genital-related issues?
- How do you think your age has affected how providers care for you?
- Do you have associated medical conditions that you think affect the way providers care for you?

Dermatology experiences

- Are there any experiences unique to dermatology that have been difficult for you (skin examination, talking about sexually transmitted diseases, and so forth)?
- How do you feel about total body skin examinations? Genital examinations?
- If you could let dermatology providers know anything about what you need in terms of good care, what would it be?
- Any advice on how to approach a patient? Connect with a patient? Make them feel comfortable?
- Would it make you more comfortable if you could just meet the dermatologist first before having to subject yourself to a full skin examination?
- How can providers best determine how to refer to your anatomy?
- Are there any impediments to a skin examination that providers should be aware of (chest binders and so forth)? If so, how can they best address these extra considerations to provide appropriate quality of care but also still be respectful? This is their PRIORITY.
- Would having an LGBTQ dermatologist or nurse present make you more comfortable with a skin check?
- Anything else that would help me to best work with you?

programs can have important formal and informal effects on the shaping of residency experiences, the tone and priorities of clinical settings, and the diversity of medical staff.

Outside of the institution, such programs also telegraph important messages to potential constituencies. They can assist with the recruitment of a more diverse medical staff and medical student population. They project a welcoming message, and they integrate LGBTQ health into the mission of the hospital, rather than portraying it as an add-on to the main purpose of the institution. Most importantly, such a program conveys a similarly welcoming message to LGBTQ-identifying patients and provides them with a practical contact point for seeking care. Patients 1 and 4, for example, found their provider at the University of Pennsylvania through the hospital's LGBTQ Health Program Web site. In scaling such programs to their own needs, smaller practices also could benefit from these positive internal and external effects.

EFFECTIVE PATIENT ENGAGEMENT

The authors encourage providers to consciously think of the first few patient meetings as a process of creating space for building the relationship with the patient, rather than expecting it to generate in a single meeting. With this focus, remain open and assume nothing about the patient's identity. Understand that information is likely to be forthcoming at certain points, and remain cognizant of the fact that patients will reveal different elements of their intersectional identity as they see fit. Build an open, humble, and honest rapport with them only accelerates that process, lead to more effective dermatologic care.

Box 2 represents purely a starting point. These questions could take the form of a questionnaire or could be incorporated (in part) into a practitioner's questioning, demonstrating sensitivity and openness to the importance of identity. With these questions, however, the dermatologist should be prepared for any answer that may come, and, if the patient seems guarded at first, there is no need to force the issue. It is also important to signal to a patient (either verbally in conversation or when discussing a questionnaire) that this information is solely to help the practitioner do the job better: serve patients and their wellness to the best possible degree.

In their own introduction, practitioners also can signal their awareness of LGBTQ identity. Along with a preferred name, a practitioner also might state preferred pronouns: "Hi, I'm Dr. Gonzalez and my preferred pronouns are she/her." For some patients, this might seem insignificant or even unexpected, but for transgender or gender nonconforming patients, this could signal a level of comfort and openness that significantly expedites the construction of doctor-patient rapport. Regardless of a patient's specific identity, it demonstrates a level of cultural competence and humility that sets the tone for all future interactions.

Also remember: mistakes happen to everyone. Even the most experienced equity and inclusion professionals will misspeak, lapse into an assumption, or misgender a patient. This is not a moment for a self-focused response, nervousness or embarrassment. Keep the perspective centered on the patient and on the patient's well-being. Recognize and acknowledge a mistake and work to ensure to not make it again. This response demonstrates a level of concern and self-awareness that signals a real interest in patients and their health.

SUMMARY

The authors hope that, reflecting on the perspectives of these patients, it is clear that dermatologists and clinical teams have an opportunity to reframe their approaches to LGBTQ patients, and, more fundamentally, to reexamine the ways in which practitioners can effectively engage with the complexity of human identity. In many ways, dermatology shares the imperatives of education, law, and other professional fields, to better serve LGBTQ-identifying individuals. The stakes are high for dermatology patients, and, when treating conditions like HPV, HIV, and cancer, effective and unbiased patient engagement can dramatically affect the quality of health care for a patient. The patient profiles represented in this article demonstrate how prioritizing self-reflection and injecting empathy into engagement with patients can fundamentally shift the patient experience and improve the quality of care.

When working with LGBTQ patients, in particular, it is incumbent on a provider to understand the disproportionately great societal and psychological threats that these patients face. It also is important that a practice provides consistent, inclusive, and nonjudgmental opportunities to empower clinical staff to pursue goals of cultural competence, cultural humility, and the recognition of intersectional identity. The authors' examination shows that prioritizing durable, internal expertise can be an effective step in this direction.

For the dermatology team, the authors also hope that this reflection has illuminated some of the unique structural elements of dermatologic practice that can define LGBTQ patient experiences. In certain cases, the focus on cancer care and cosmetic treatment, along with the social stigma that accompanies the physical manifestations of certain dermatologic conditions, has inhibited the widespread implementation of inclusive norms for LGBTQ patient populations. The authors argue that, given the specific needs of LGBTQ patients, dermatologists have an opportunity and a responsibility to take a leading role in the development of increasingly effective clinical practices for this patient population.

DISCLOSURE

None of the authors has any commercial or financial conflicts of interest.

REFERENCES

1. Charny JW, Kovarik CL. LGBT access to health care: a dermatologist's role in building a therapeutic relationship. Cutis 2017;99(4):228–9.
2. "LGBT Health Program – Penn Medicine." – Penn Medicine, 2018. Available at: www.pennmedicine.org/for-patients-and-visitors/find-a-program-or-service/lgbt-health. Accessed April 1, 2019.
3. (Un)equal care for all? Dermatology World 2018; 46–8.
4. Ufomata E, Eckstrand K, Hasley P, et al. Comprehensive internal medicine residency curriculum on primary care of patients who identify as LGBT. LGBT Health 2018;5(6):375–80.
5. Chapman EN, Kaatz A, Carnes M. Physicians and implicit bias: how doctors may unwittingly perpetuate health care disparities. J Gen Intern Med 2013;28(11):1504–10.
6. Saha S, Beach MC, Cooper LA. Patient centeredness, cultural competence and healthcare quality. J Natl Med Assoc 2008;100(11):1275–85.
7. Crenshaw K. Mapping the margins: intersectionality, identity politics, and violence against women of color. Stanford Law Rev 1991;43(6):1241–99.
8. LGBTQ Youth, June 2017. Available at: https://www.cdc.gov/lgbthealth/youth.htm, Centers for Disease Control and Prevention. Accessed April 15, 2019.
9. Welcoming schools program. Human Rights Campaign Foundation; 2019. Available at: http://www.welcomingschools.org. Accessed April 15, 2019.
10. Shlasko D, Hofius K. Trans allyship workbook: building skills to support trans people in our lives. Brattleboro (VT): Think Again Training; 2017.
11. Tervalon M, Murray-García J. Cultural humility versus cultural competence: a critical distinction in defining physician training outcomes in multicultural education. J Health Care Poor Underserved 1998;9(2): 117–25.
12. Ruud M. Cultural humility in the care of individuals who are lesbian, gay, bisexual, transgender, or queer. Nurs Womens Health 2018;22(3):255–63.
13. Montenery S, Jones A, Perry N, et al. Cultural competence in nursing faculty: a journey, not a destination. J Prof Nurs 2013;29(6):e51–7.
14. Butler M, McCreedy E, Schwer N, et al. Improving cultural competence to reduce health disparities. Rockville (MD): Agency for Healthcare Research and Quality (US); 2016 (Comparative Effectiveness Reviews, No. 170.) 3, Lesbian, Gay, Bisexual, and Transgender Populations. Available at: https://www.ncbi.nlm.nih.gov/books/NBK361118/.
15. Mortensen GL, Larsen HK. The quality of life of patients with genital warts: a qualitative study. BMC Public Health 2010;10:113.
16. Ginsberg B, Calderon M, Seminara N, et al. A potential role for the dermatologist in the physical transformation of transgender people: a survey of attitudes and practices within the transgender community. J Am Acad Dermatol 2016;74(2):303–8.
17. "LGBT Health Initiative." – UCLA Health, 2019. Available at: https://www.uclahealth.org/lgbtq/our-expert-team. Accessed April 1, 2019.

Update on Medical Education, Insurance Coverage, and Health Care Policy for Lesbian, Gay, Bisexual, Transgender, Questioning, Intersexual, and Asexual Patients

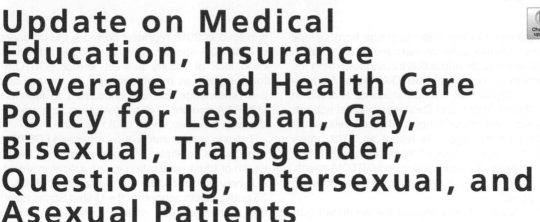

Tien Viet Nguyen, MD

KEYWORDS

- Medical education • Insurance coverage • Health care policy • LGBTQIA

KEY POINTS

- There are important gaps in LGBTQIA knowledge, clinical competency, and cultural sensitivity, as well as attitudes among health care professionals, medical educators, and those in the public and insurance policy sectors.
- These are not only professional deficiencies but also perpetuate discrimination, limit access to health care, and lead to poor health outcomes.
- Research supports the notion that acquiring skills and knowledge through dedicated training programs leads to more compassionate and competent care for LGBTQIA patients.

INTRODUCTION

The need to increase training for health care professionals and support staff to provide competent, sensitive, and compassionate care for lesbian, gay, bisexual, transgender, questioning, intersexual, and asexual (LGBTQIA) individuals has gathered momentum in the past few decades. This is rightly so because according to the Institute of Medicine's 2011 report of LGBTQIA health disparity and research gaps, this unique population continues to face significant discrimination and health care barriers.[1] In 2014, The Association of American Medical Colleges (AAMC) took a big step in acknowledging issues encountered by LGBTQIA patients and provided institutional guidance for change in a document titled "Implementing Curricular and Institutional Climate Changes to Improve Health Care for Individuals Who Are LGBT, Gender Nonconforming (GNC), or Born with Differences of Sex Development (DSD)."[2] This article focuses on deficiencies in medical education and research, insurance coverage, and health care policy for LGBTQIA patients, and also highlights a few examples of successful initiatives to fix them. The term "sexual and gender minority" may be used interchangeably with "LGBTQIA." Both terms are meant to include the entire spectrum of sexual and gender identities.

MEDICAL EDUCATION AND RESEARCH GAPS REGARDING HEALTH IN LESBIAN, GAY, BISEXUAL, TRANSGENDER, QUESTIONING, INTERSEXUAL, AND ASEXUAL PATIENTS

The deficiency in providing compassionate, multidisciplinary care to address the needs of sexual

Bellevue Dermatology Clinic, 1810 116th Avenue Northeast #100, Bellevue, WA 98004, USA
E-mail address: letien62nguyen@gmail.com

Dermatol Clin 38 (2020) 201–207
https://doi.org/10.1016/j.det.2019.10.004

and gender minority patients stems from several issues. One foundational area needing rectification is the inadequate education/training regarding the provision of competent LGBTQIA health. A survey in 2011 found that medical students enrolled at 132 United States and Canadian medical schools only received about 5 hours of LGBT-related didactics on average.[3] As recent as 2012, many United States academic institutions still report lacking or insufficient training on LGBTQIA health, with the majority expressing interest in addressing this issue.[4]

This issue extends beyond the American borders. In a single-centered survey in the United Kingdom, approximately 85% of medical students across all years of education reported lack of confidence and competence in caring for LGBTQIA patients.[5] Even though the respondents held positive attitudes toward the LGBTQIA community, they lacked confidence in performing crucial information-gathering functions such as clarifying gender pronouns or querying patients regarding their sexual identity. Other elements of the patient-provider encounters were also reported to be deficient, including providing resources and discussing domestic abuse with LGBTQIA patients.

LGBTQIA patients also echo discrimination and a lack of provider knowledge as important barriers to receiving good care. A United States–based survey of about 7000 transgender individuals in 2010 illuminated 3 key shortcomings of our current medical system.[6] First, 19% of survey respondents cited their gender identity as the reason they were refused care.[6] Second, 28% reported experiencing verbal harassment in the medical setting, with 2% reporting having encountered violence in physicians' offices.[6] Third, lack of provider knowledge was rampant: 50% reported having to teach their providers about competent care for transgender patients.[6]

At the moment, many specialties do not require sexual and gender minority–specific content as part of their graduate medical education. Here, emergency medicine and psychiatry are discussed as case studies for no particular reason except the availability of published data. The 2011 curricular guidelines for emergency medicine residency training did not include topics relevant to LGBTQIA health.[7] A recent survey study found that only 26% of the 124 United States–based emergency medicine residency directors reported having presented a lecture on LGBTQIA health, with an average didactic time of 45 minutes.[8]

Psychiatry residency training faces a similar problem. Approximately half of the 72 United States–based adult psychiatry program directors surveyed in 2018 reported no more than 5 hours of LGBTQIA-specific training. Program directors cited lack of faculty interest and/or LGBTQIA-topic experts as major barriers.[9] To the author's best knowledge, current endeavors to increase LGBTQIA content in dermatology training are under way; however, more could be done.

Training and research gaps regarding LGBTQIA care spans multiple health professions. Public health graduate education is one salient example. A survey completed by 102 department chairs of 35 public health schools in the United States found that a meager 9% offered courses regarding LGBTQIA health beyond HIV/AIDS.[10] Eighteen percent of the respondents were aware of their own faculty, who researched non-HIV/AIDS LGBTQIA health issues.[10] Furthermore, only 10% were aware of completed doctorate theses advancing public health knowledge and care of the sexual and gender minority community.[10]

Counselors and psychologists play a significant role in LGBTQIA health care by helping patients cope with social stigmatization, self-esteem issues, and psychological distress related to their health needs. They, too, have echoed the need for better preparation to provide competent care and counseling to LGBTQIA individuals.[11] Future research should concentrate on assessing LGBTQIA educational research gaps in other aspects of health care not mentioned heretofore to guide more comprehensive reform.

PROGRESS IN MEDICAL EDUCATION AND TRAINING OPPORTUNITIES REGARDING HEALTHCARE FOR LESBIAN, GAY, BISEXUAL, TRANSGENDER, QUESTIONING, INTERSEXUAL, AND ASEXUAL PATIENTS
Training at the Undergraduate Health Professions Level

In terms of increasing awareness and instilling cultural sensitivity for medical students, a few efforts are worth mentioning. The eQuality Project at the University of Louisville aims to lay the foundation for a multidisciplinary systematic approach to competent care for LGBTQIA patients.[12] Preproject and postproject assessments showed an increase in student interest toward interprofessional teamwork. After the course, the participants were also more likely to consider systematic and social factors influencing health disparities in the LGBTQIA community.[12]

Leaders in LGBTQIA health education have employed the same standardized-patient-based method with success in honing important clinical skills, such as taking an inclusive medical history free of implicit biases.[13] At the Johns Hopkins

University School of Medicine, first-year medical students demonstrated that after clinical modules with standardized patients, 92% felt more prepared to elicit a thorough sexual history from LGBTQIA patients.[14] Knowledge gain on behalf of the trainees also occurred, whereby 90% of them were able to define the term "transgender" correctly after the training.[14] Training assessments helped identify unmet needs for this group: to educate students regarding social stigma and health care barriers faced by LGBTQIA patients.[14]

Institution-wide lectures and courses may provide benefits to students of various health professions, not just medical students. One such example is the Transgender Health Course at the University of California, San Francisco (UCSF).[15] Developed by transgender medicine faculty experts and student leaders, the program offered convenient lunch-hour lectures to students in the medicine, pharmacy, dentistry, advanced practice nursing, and physical therapy schools at UCSF. The students who took the precourse and postcourse surveys exhibited an increase in key knowledge domains in transgender medicine and reduced transphobia.[15,16] Interestingly, half of the course instructors were themselves transgender—whether this contributed to the program's success is unknown. Student leaders played a pivotal role in developing the program's content by providing the instructors with the course objectives.[15]

Training at the Graduate Medical Education Level

At the graduate medical education level, the creation of an LGBTQIA primary care tract for internal medicine residents at the University of Pittsburgh Health System has proved to be beneficial. Precurricular and postcurricular assessments among the 153 residents across all years of training showed a statistically significant increase in knowledge base with regard to LGBTQIA health.[17] The curriculum also boosted the residents' confidence in their ability to implement gender-neutral practices in their future practices.[17]

On a larger scale, the Penn Medicine Program for LGBT Health aimed to educate students, residents, and faculty members regarding LGBTQIA health as well as to increase visibility of the institution's LGBTQIA community. The Program resulted in a series of institution-wide lectures, networking events, and community-oriented activities.[18] The creators of this program reported their institutional climate, planning process, and structure as well as lessons learned from its implementation. This detailed report may serve as a blueprint for other

institutions to take on their own LGBTQIA health education initiatives.

Several studies have shown that a diverse faculty with LGBTQIA members may positively influence training programs. A survey by Moll and colleagues[8] on emergency medicine residency directors found that 64.2% of the 124 programs had LGBT faculty. The presence of LGBT faculty and previous education on LGBT health were found to correlate positively with a desire for more training.[8] By contrast, Hirschtritt and colleagues[9] identified lack of topic-expert faculty as a crucial barrier to adequate training among psychiatry residency programs. These studies emphasize the importance of recruiting faculty members from sexual and gender minority backgrounds or those who are LGBTQIA health experts.

Training Opportunities for the Health Care Workforce

Several studies on "interdisciplinary" LGBTQIA training have shown positive results. "Interdisciplinary" refers to the training of an entire team working in the same department or setting, including those in medicine, nursing, nutrition, social work, and psychology. For example, an online training module aimed at increasing LGBTQIA cultural competency at geriatric long-term care facilities was successful at increasing staff members' knowledge.[19] Similarly, an interdisciplinary curriculum in adolescent medicine helped learners gain confidence in caring for LGBTQIA youth, provide local and national resources, and self-assess their skills for further development.[20]

In oncology, a Web-based training model was developed with input from LGBTQIA cancer survivors, cultural competency experts, oncologists, and Web and instructional designers.[21] This project is awaiting field validation. Meanwhile, researchers have assessed the effects of cultural competency training administered to a mixed sample of emergency medicine physicians, nurse practitioners, nurses, and unit secretaries.[22] A staggering 85% of the staff had not received any prior LGBTQIA health education. Three to 5 months after the intervention, the team demonstrated a significant increase in collective knowledge and skills in caring for LGBTQIA patients.[22] They also reported more openness and awareness of oppression faced by the LGBTQIA community.[22]

Beyond the individual workplace, multidisciplinary conferences are now offered nationwide. One such conference is the LGBT Healthcare Workforce Conference, a joint effort among several health care organizations.[23] The first annual conference in New York was attended by 250 individuals, including high school and college students, graduate students, and health care professionals.[23] Topics presented at the conference ranged from professional leadership development to research funding and LGBTQIA public policy.[23] The conference also included mentoring sessions, which foster professional relationships and career development for the LGBTQIA-focused health care workforce.

HEALTH CARE POLICY AND INSURANCE COVERAGE FOR LESBIAN, GAY, BISEXUAL, TRANSGENDER, QUESTIONING, INTERSEXUAL, AND ASEXUAL INDIVIDUALS

At the moment, the Center for Medicare and Medicaid Services (CMS) does not cover for services related to sex reassignment surgeries (SRS).[24] With approximately 1.4 million adults in the United States identifying as transgender in 2016, many aging transgender individuals will depend on Medicare for health services.[25] Although routine care and hormonal therapy for gender dysphoria are covered by Medicare, transgender patients usually require surgeries to avoid the burdens of mental health disorders, and even self-harm. Lack of health care options may prompt some transgender patients to seek help from low-cost, illicit surgery centers operating in and outside the United States, sometimes with devastating outcomes.

The US Department of Veterans Affairs (VA) also denies coverage for SRS, with language indicating a belief that SRS is not part of standard general practice for gender dysphoria.[26] This is a major shortcoming in their policy toward former LGBTQIA military and service members, and needs to change. Nevertheless, the VA has made major strides in other aspects, such as the creation of the LGBT Program within the Office for Diversity and Inclusion. They have also added gender identity protections to the Equal Employment Opportunity Commission protections.[27–29]

There is a paucity of data on how the repeal of the "Don't Ask, Don't Tell" policy in 2011 has affected health care for active-duty military members identifying as LGBTQIA. A single-center study found that only 5% of primary care providers in the military inquired about their patients' same-sex activity.[30] One-third of the respondents had received prior training on LGBTQIA health while many desired clearer guidance from the Department of Defense regarding screening and documentation of military members' sexual behavior.[30]

Coverage of SRS for transgender individuals with private insurances still faces major challenges, especially in the adolescent LGBTQIA population. A single-center chart review found that insurance companies reimbursed for hormonal therapy in only 8 of the 27 adolescent transgender patients.[31] One patient's family absorbed the out-of-pocket cost of therapy.[31] Lack of insurance coverage effectively denied the remaining 18 patients of much-needed treatment for their gender dysphoria. The investigators made a poignant case for the shortsightedness of these insurance companies. After examining 79 transgender patient records, they found a 92% rate of mental health disorders, 74% rate of suicidal ideation, and a 55% rate of self-harm and suicidal behaviors in this cohort.[31] Managing these conditions will likely be more costly than reimbursing the transgender patients' identity-affirming therapies.

Several professional organizations have recognized that medical intervention is a benefit that outweighs possible risks.[31,32] To ease concerns about escalating costs, the American Medical Association suggested that appropriate treatments for gender dysphoria might actually be cost-saving to the health care system.[33] Anecdotal evidence exists to support this claim. For example, the City of San Francisco discovered that transgender services in their employee health plan were less costly than previously thought. Therefore, the city removed surcharges related to these benefits in 2006.[33,34]

LEGISLATIVE STEPS TOWARD BETTER HEALTH CARE FOR LESBIAN, GAY, BISEXUAL, TRANSGENDER, QUESTIONING, INTERSEXUAL, AND ASEXUAL INDIVIDUALS

A few important legal tools can be used to champion the coverage of medical care for the sexual and gender minority community. The 2009 federal bill "Ending LGBT Health Disparities Act" aimed to protect patients against discrimination based on their sexual orientation and gender identity by Medicare, Medicaid, and Children's Health Insurance programs.[33,35] The Equal Employment Opportunity Commission ruled in 2012 that the Civil Rights Act's Title VII prohibitions against sex-based discrimination at work also apply to transgender individuals.[36] In the same year, the Department of Health and Human Services clarified that discrimination based on gender identity is part of the ban on sex discrimination within the Patient Protection and Affordable Care Act.[33]

In 2010, former President Barack Obama signed into law a health care reform bill that prevents insurers from labeling being transgender as a pre-existing health condition. This portion of the law became enforceable in 2014. An update is needed to understand how it has affected transgender individuals with respect to health insurance access.

SUMMARY

There are important gaps in LGBTQIA knowledge, clinical competency, and cultural sensitivity, as well as attitudes among health care professionals, medical educators, and those in the public and insurance policy sectors. These are not only professional deficiencies but also perpetuate discrimination, limit access to health care, and lead to poor health outcomes. Research supports the notion that acquiring skills and knowledge through dedicated training programs leads to more compassionate and competent care for LGBTQIA patients.

Educational opportunities may take varying forms. As discussed in this chapter, they range from early institutionalized curricula in health professional schools, graduate medical training programs, interdisciplinary courses, institutional initiatives, and continuing medical education activities to nationwide health conferences. Finally, LGBTQIA patients, their families, and allies will likely play a major role in prioritizing education, research, and policy initiatives regarding LGBTQIA health care in the future.[37,38]

RESOURCES

National government and nongovernment programs to develop interdisciplinary training for health care providers and staff[39]:

- Gay & Lesbian Medical Association (GLMA)— Health Professionals Advancing LGBT Equality: www.glma.org
- National LGBT Cancer Network: www.cancer-network.org
- The Fenway Institute—National LGBT Health Education Center: www.lgbthealtheducation.org
- Substance Abuse and Mental Health Services Administration (SAMHSA)—LGBT Training Curricula for Behavioral Health and Primary Care Practitioners: www.samhsa.gov/behavioral-health-equity/lgbt/curricula
- US Department of Veterans Affairs—Patient Care Services & LGBT Veteran Training: www.patientcare.va.gov/LGBT/LGBT_Veteran_Training.asp
- Whitman-Walker Health: www.whitman-walker.org/service/community-health/mautner-project

Examples of academic institutions and medical centers with LGBT multidisciplinary care and educational programs:

- Center of Excellence for Transgender Health—University of California, San Francisco: www.transhealth.ucsf.edu
- Integrated Transgender Program—University of Colorado Health: https://www.uchealth.org/services/diabetes-endocrinology-care/uchealth-integrated-transgender-program/
- LGBT Healthy Policy and Practice Program—George Washington University: https://lgbt.columbian.gwu.edu
- Center for LGBT Health Research certificate program at the Graduate School of Public Health—University of Pittsburgh: www.lgbthlres.pitt.edu

DISCLOSURE

No relevant conflict of interest to disclose.

REFERENCES

1. US Institute of Medicine. Committee on lesbian, gay, bisexual, and transgender health issues and research gaps and opportunities. The health of lesbian, gay, bisexual, and transgender people: building a foundation for better understanding. Washington (DC): National Academies Press; 2011. Available at: http://www.ncbi.nlm.nih.gov/books/NBK64806/. Accessed May 11, 2019.
2. Association of American Medical Colleges. Implementing curricular and institutional climate changes to improve health care for individuals who are LGBT, gender nonconforming, or born with DSD. Washington, DC: AAMC; 2014.
3. Obedin-Maliver J, Goldsmith ES, Stewart L, et al. Lesbian, gay, bisexual, and transgender-related content in undergraduate medical education. JAMA 2011;306(9):971–7.
4. Khalili J, Leung LB, Diamant AL. Finding the perfect doctor: identifying lesbian, gay, bisexual, and transgender-competent physicians. Am J Public Health 2015;105(6):1114–9.
5. Parameshwaran V, Cockbain BC, Hillyard M, et al. Is the lack of specific lesbian, gay, bisexual, transgender and queer/questioning (LGBTQ) health care education in medical school a cause for concern? Evidence from a survey of knowledge and practice among UK medical students. J Homosex 2017;64(3):367–81.
6. Grant JM, Mottet LA, Tanis J, et al. National transgender discrimination survey report on health and health care. Washington, DC: National Center for Transgender Equality; 2010.

7. 2011 EM Model Review Task Force, Perina DG, Brunett CP, Caro DA, et al. The 2011 model of the clinical practice of emergency medicine. Acad Emerg Med 2012;19(7):e19–40.

8. Moll J, Krieger P, Moreno-Walton L, et al. The prevalence of lesbian, gay, bisexual, and transgender health education and training in emergency medicine residency programs: what do we know? Acad Emerg Med 2014;21(5):608–11.

9. Hirschtritt ME, Noy G, Haller E, et al. LGBT-specific education in general psychiatry residency programs: a survey of program directors. Acad Psychiatry 2019;43(1):41–5.

10. Corliss HL, Shankle MD, Moyer MB. Research, curricula, and resources related to lesbian, gay, bisexual, and transgender health in US schools of public health. Am J Public Health 2007;97(6):1023–7.

11. Bidell MP. Examining school counseling students' multicultural and sexual orientation competencies through a cross-specialization comparison. J Couns Dev 2012;90(2):200–7.

12. Leslie KF, Steinbock S, Simpson R, et al. Interprofessional LGBT health equity education for early learners. MedEdPORTAL 2017;13:10551.

13. Mayfield JJ, Ball EM, Tillery KA, et al. Beyond men, women, or both: a comprehensive, LGBTQ-inclusive, implicit-bias-aware, standardized-patient-based sexual history taking curriculum. MedEdPORTAL 2017;13:10634.

14. Bakhai N, Ramos J, Gorfinkle N, et al. Introductory learning of inclusive sexual history taking: an E-lecture, standardized patient case, and facilitated debrief. MedEdPORTAL 2016;12:10520.

15. Braun HM, Garcia-Grossman IR, Quiñones-Rivera A, et al. Outcome and impact evaluation of a transgender health course for health profession students. LGBT Health 2017;4(1):55–61.

16. Nagoshi JL, Adams KA, Terrell HK, et al. Gender differences in correlates of homophobia and transphobia. Sex Roles 2008;59(7–8):521–31.

17. Ufomata E, Eckstrand KL, Hasley P, et al. Comprehensive internal medicine residency curriculum on primary care of patients who identify as LGBT. LGBT Health 2018;5(6):375–80.

18. Yehia BR, Calder D, Flesch JD, et al. Advancing LGBT health at an academic medical center: a case study. LGBT Health 2015;2(4):362–6.

19. Donaldson W, Smith HM, Parrish BP. Serving all who served: piloting an online tool to support cultural competency with LGBT U.S. Military veterans in long-term care. Clin Gerontol 2019;42(2):185–91.

20. Calzo JP, Melchiono M, Richmond TK, et al. Lesbian, gay, bisexual, and transgender adolescent health: an interprofessional case discussion. MedEdPORTAL 2017;13:10615.

21. Seay J, Hicks A, Markham MJ, et al. Developing a web-based LGBT cultural competency training for oncologists: The COLORS training. Patient Educ Couns 2019;102(5):984–9.

22. Bristol S, Kostelec T, MacDonald R. Improving emergency health care workers' knowledge, competency, and attitudes toward lesbian, gay, bisexual, and transgender patients through interdisciplinary cultural competency training. J Emerg Nurs 2018;44(6):632–9.

23. Sánchez NF, Sánchez JP, Lunn MR, et al. First annual LGBT health workforce conference: empowering our health workforce to better serve LGBT communities. LGBT Health 2014;1(1):62–5.

24. Chapter 1: coverage determinations, part 2: section 140.3: transsexual surgery. In: Medicare National Coverage Determination (NCD) Manual.

25. Flores AR, Herman JL, Gates GJ, et al. How many adults identify as transgender in the United States? Los Angeles (CA): The Williams Institute; 2016.

26. Veterans Health Administration: Medical benefits package. 38 CFR 17.38.

27. Veterans Health Administration: LGBT Program. Available at: http://www.diversity.va.gov/programs/lgbt.aspx.

28. USDVA Office of Diversity and Inclusion. USDVA ODI Secretary's Equal Employment Opportunity (EEO), diversity and inclusion, and No FEAR policy statement. Washington, DC: ODI; 2012.

29. Veterans Health Administration. VHA Directive 2011-024: providing health care for transgender and intersex veterans. Washington, DC: VHA; 2011.

30. Rerucha CM, Runser LA, Ee JS, et al. Military healthcare providers' knowledge and comfort regarding the medical care of active duty lesbian, gay, and bisexual patients. LGBT Health 2018;5(1):86–90.

31. Nahata L, Quinn GP, Caltabellotta NM, et al. Mental health concerns and insurance denials among transgender adolescents. LGBT Health 2017;4(3):188–93.

32. Murad MH, Elamin MB, Garcia MZ, et al. Hormonal therapy and sex reassignment: a systematic review and meta-analysis of quality of life and psychosocial outcomes. Clin Endocrinol (Oxf) 2010;72(2):214–31.

33. Stroumsa D. The state of transgender health care: policy, law, and medical frameworks. Am J Public Health 2014;104(3):e31–8.

34. City and County of San Francisco. San Francisco City and County transgender health benefit. San Francisco (CA): San Francisco Human Rights Commission; 2007.

35. H.R. 3001 - Ending LGBT Health Disparities Act. 2010 2009.

36. Macy v Holder. Appeal No. 0120120821. Agency No. ATF-2011-00751. 2012.

37. Logie CH, Lys C. The process of developing a community-based research agenda with lesbian, gay, bisexual, transgender and queer youth in the Northwest Territories, Canada. Int J Circumpolar Health 2015;74(1):28188.

38. Noonan EJ, Sawning S, Combs R, et al. Engaging the transgender community to improve medical education and prioritize healthcare initiatives. Teach Learn Med 2018;30(2):119–32.

39. Bidell MP, Stepleman LM. An interdisciplinary approach to lesbian, gay, bisexual, and transgender clinical competence, professional training, and ethical care: introduction to the special issue. J Homosex 2017;64(10):1305–29.

Skin Cancer and Skin Cancer Risk Factors in Sexual and Gender Minorities

Dustin H. Marks, BS[a], Sarah Tuttleton Arron, MD, PhD[b],
Matthew Mansh, MD[c],*

KEYWORDS

- Skin cancer • Sexual minority • Gender minority • Indoor tanning • Alcohol use • Tobacco use
- Human immunodeficiency virus • Human papillomavirus

KEY POINTS

- Sexual and gender minority patients have unique risk factors that may increase their risk for developing keratinocyte carcinomas and melanoma.
- Sexual minority men are significantly more likely than heterosexual men to report a history of skin cancer, likely in part owing to increased ultraviolet radiation exposure through indoor tanning and outdoor sun exposure.
- Use of estrogen hormone therapy may place transwomen and other gender minorities at increased risk for melanoma.
- High rates of alcohol and tobacco use and concomitant infection with human immunodeficiency virus and human papillomavirus represent other potential skin cancer risk factors among sexual and gender minorities.
- Future research is critical to develop appropriate screening practices and tailored interventions to decrease skin cancer and associated risk factors in sexual and gender minorities.

INTRODUCTION

Skin cancer is the most common cancer in the United States and affects 1 in 5 Americans over their lifetime. Skin cancer treatments impose a significant economic burden on the US health care system, costing an average of $8.1 billion annually.[1] The incidence of both keratinocyte carcinomas and melanoma have increased significantly, with rates of cutaneous squamous cell carcinoma (cSCC) alone increasing 263% between the time periods 1976 to 1984 and 2000 to 2010. This is likely owing to increasing UV radiation (UVR) exposure from both natural sunlight and indoor tanning devices.[1–5] In 2014, the Surgeon General released a *Call to Action to Prevent Skin Cancer* to address the increasing impact of skin cancer-related morbidity, mortality, and cost in the United States.[6] Specifically, it called for increased efforts to identify at-risk populations and increase awareness of and develop effective public policy and prevention efforts aimed to reduce preventable risk factors such as UVR.[6–8]

Emerging evidence suggests that sexual and gender minorities (SGM)—especially sexual minority men—may have higher rates of skin cancer and unique skin cancer risk factors and related

a Department of Dermatology, Massachusetts General Hospital, 50 Staniford Street, Suite 200, Boston, MA 02114, USA; b Department of Dermatology, University of California, San Francisco, 1701 Divisadero Street, 3rd Floor, San Francisco, CA 94143-0316, USA; c Department of Dermatology, University of Minnesota, 516 Delaware Street Southeast, Mail Code 98, Phillips-Wangensteen Building, Suite 4-240, Minneapolis, MN 55455, USA
* Corresponding author.
E-mail address: mansh@umn.edu

Dermatol Clin 38 (2020) 209–218
https://doi.org/10.1016/j.det.2019.10.005

behaviors. Although clinicians and public health researchers have become increasingly aware of the health care needs of SGM populations over the last several decades, the National Institutes of Health only recently designated SGM as an official health disparities population alongside racial/ethnic minorities, socioeconomically disadvantaged populations, and underserved rural populations.[9,10] The federal government's public health agenda, Healthy People 2020, aims to eliminate SGM health disparities. It is critical that dermatologists are aware of the relevant health care problems experienced by SGM people to achieve this objective. In this review, we focus on skin cancer, skin cancer risk factors, and related behaviors in SGM.

TERMINOLOGY

SGM is an umbrella term that includes lesbian, gay, bisexual, and transgender individuals in addition to other persons whose sexual orientation, gender identity, and/or gender expression differ from traditional, societal, cultural, or physiologic norms.[9] *Gender identify* refers to an individual's self-perception as male, female, a combination of both, or neither. *Gender expression* represents the external manifestations or outward manner in which a person displays their gender (eg, clothing, speech patterns, mannerisms). *Transgender* serves as the term to describe a person whose gender identity or gender expression differs from the sex that they were assigned at birth, which is typically based on external genital anatomy. More specifically, a *transman* is a person who identifies as a man but was assigned a female sex at birth, whereas a *transwoman* is a person who identifies as a woman and was assigned a male sex at birth. Separate from gender identity is *sexual orientation*, which describes a person's enduring pattern of emotional, romantic, and/or sexual attraction to persons of the opposite, same, or other gender/sex (eg, lesbian, gay, straight).[11]

SEXUAL MINORITIES
Skin Cancer

Sexual minority men may be a high-risk population for developing skin cancer.[12] In a cross-sectional study using data from the 2001, 2003, 2005, and 2009 California Health Interview Surveys (CHISs) and the 2013 National Health Interview Survey (NHIS), sexual minority men compared with heterosexual men were found to have an increased odds of reporting a history of skin cancer (2001–2005 CHISs: 4.3% vs 2.7%, adjusted odds ratio [aOR], 1.56; $P = .002$; 2013 NHIS: 6.7% vs 3.2%; aOR, 2.13; $P = .02$), including nonmelanoma skin cancer (2001–2005 CHISs: 2.9% vs 2.0%; aOR, 1.44; $P = .04$) and melanoma (2001–2005 CHISs: 1.1% vs 0.6%; aOR, 1.68; $P = .02$). In contrast, sexual minority women compared with heterosexual women were found to have a significantly lower odds of reporting a history of nonmelanoma skin cancer (2001–2005 CHISs: 1.1% vs 1.8%; aOR, 0.56; $P = .008$), but no differences in rates of melanoma.[12] Although other known skin cancer risk factors, such as family history, Fitzpatrick skin type, and/or geographic location, may vary by sexual orientation, the authors concluded that uncontrolled behaviors related to UVR exposure were most likely to account for the significant differences in rates of skin cancer found between sexual minority and heterosexual men. This study does have notable limitations, including use of self-reported data that were not adjudicated by medical record review, and further research is needed to validate the association between sexual orientation and skin cancer.

Indoor Tanning

Considering all risk factors, UVR exposure—from both sunlight and artificial sources—represents one of the most preventable cause of skin cancer. Although eliminating outdoor sun exposure may be more difficult for certain individuals (eg, those with occupational exposure in the construction or agricultural sectors), use of indoor tanning devices is entirely avoidable.[6,13] Classified as carcinogenic to humans (group 1) by the International Agency for Research on Cancer, UVR-emitting tanning devices including sun/tanning lamps, beds, and booths are classified in the same category as the alpha- and beta-particle emitters that were released after the Chernobyl accident.[14] A number of systematic reviews and meta-analyses have supported the association of indoor tanning with an increased risk of both keratinocyte carcinomas and melanoma.[15–17] Specifically, any use of indoor tanning before the age of 35 is associated with a 75% increased risk of developing melanoma.[15] There is a strong dose-dependent relationship between melanoma risk and frequency of indoor tanning, because those with melanoma compared with those without melanoma were more likely to report more hours ($P<.0001$), more years ($P<.006$), and more sessions ($P = .0002$) of indoor tanning.[18] In addition, any use of indoor tanning is associated with a 67% and 29% higher risk of developing cSCC and basal cell carcinoma (BCC), respectively.[16,17]

Most epidemiologic studies investigating indoor tanning have focused on young, non-Hispanic white females.[6,19–21] Specifically, 30% and 25% of non-Hispanic white female high school students and young adults, respectively, report indoor tanning at least once in the last year. Among young women, indoor tanning is closely associated with impaired body image, depression, and appearance concerns, demonstrating that psychological and social factors represent motivators of UVR exposure.[22–24] Sexual minority men are also more likely to have body image issues, report greater self-objectification, more frequent appearance-based social comparisons, and demonstrate higher rates of eating disorders and body dysmorphic disorder when compared with heterosexual men.[25–29] These factors likely predispose sexual minority men to engage in indoor tanning.

Prevalence of indoor tanning

Sexual minority men report higher rates of indoor tanning than heterosexual men, although the existing literature presents somewhat conflicting results on rates of indoor tanning among sexual minority women.[12,30–32] Among adults, sexual minority men compared with heterosexual men have been found to have a significantly increased odds of reporting indoor tanning in the last year (2009 CHISs: 7.4% vs 1.5%; aOR; 5.80, $P<.001$; 2013 NHIS: 5.1% vs 1.6%; aOR, 3.16; $P<.001$).[12] Further studies have confirmed these findings, including that gay and bisexual men compared with heterosexual men report higher odds of both any indoor tanning (OR, 3.1 and OR, 4.5, respectively) and frequent indoor tanning (OR, 4.8 and OR, 6.5, respectively), defined as 10 or more tanning sessions in the last year.[30]

Among women, sexual minority compared with heterosexual women have been found to have significantly lower rates of indoor tanning (2009 CHISs: 2.6% vs 5.0%; aOR, 0.43; $P = .03$; 2013 NHIS: 4.2% vs 6.5%; aOR, 0.46; $P = .007$).[12] Although some studies have found no differences in rates of indoor tanning between sexual minority and heterosexual women.[30]

Among adolescents and young adults, sexual minority compared with heterosexual men are also more likely to report indoor tanning.[31,32] In a longitudinal, population-based study of adolescents, sexual minority compared with heterosexual men were significantly more likely to report indoor tanning (27.0% vs 8.6%; OR, 3.9; $P = .002$).[32] Another study found that young, black sexual minority males report the highest prevalence of indoor tanning, with rates comparable with those among white females. Although rates of indoor tanning did not differ between young heterosexual and sexual minority females among non-Hispanic white individuals, the authors did find increased rates of indoor tanning among young sexual minorities compared with heterosexual females who identified as black or Hispanic.[31]

Motivations for indoor tanning

Sexual minority men also have unique motivations for indoor tanning.[31,33] First, indoor tanning is strongly associated with a desire to improve physical appearance and body image.[23] A cross-sectional study using an online survey found that sexual minority men were more likely to engage in indoor tanning if they had darker skin tone ideals and/or a perceived skin tone that did not match their ideal.[34] Admassu and colleagues[35] conducted qualitative interviews with 48 sexual minority adult men to further understand the reasons for starting and stopping indoor tanning. Motivating factors to indoor tanning included appearance concerns (ie, achieving tanned skin) and social pressures (eg, tanning as a group activity, particularly with female friends). Concerns about skin aging and skin cancer represented the primary motivations to stop indoor tanning.[35]

Second, affect regulation represents another critical motivator of indoor tanning in sexual minority men.[31,36,37] Among cisgender individuals, the positive mood-altering effects of UV light represents a significant motivator for initiating indoor tanning and a deterrent for quitting.[33,38,39] Among sexual minority males, affect regulation has also been found to be associated with indoor tanning and future intentions to indoor tan.[37]

Finally, indoor tanning may be addictive and sexual minorities are more prone, in general, to engage in addictive behaviors. Many sexual minority individuals experience sexual minority stress—the stigma, prejudice, and discrimination toward sexual minorities that creates hostile social environments and subsequently increased psychological distress. This factor, in part, leads sexual minorities to engage in higher rates of certain addictive behaviors, such as use of tobacco, alcohol, and other substances.[36,37,40,41] Indoor tanning may also be addictive. A single-institution study of 421 college students found that 39.3% of indoor tanners met the *Diagnostics and Statistical Manual of Mental Disorders*, 4th edition, criteria for addiction, and that these individuals reported increased use of alcohol, marijuana, and other substances.[42] Thus, sexual minorities may be more susceptible to initiate and continue to engage in indoor tanning owing to its addictive nature.

Other Tanning Behaviors

Outdoor tanning, sunless tanning, and sun protection behaviors also differ by sexual orientation.[6,32,43] A cross-sectional study using data from the 2015 NHIS found that sexual minority compared with heterosexual men had increased odd of using sunless tanning products and avoiding sun exposure. Sexual minority men were also more likely to use sunscreen and seek shade, but less likely to use protective clothing (eg, long sleeves, long pants, baseball cap, or wide-brimmed hat) when outdoors and had lower overall composite sun protection scores than heterosexual men.[43] In epidemiologic studies, frequent use of sunscreen and sunless tanning have both been associated with increased outdoor sun exposure and these findings may indicate higher rates of recreational or intentional outdoor sun exposure among sexual minority men.[44,45] Outdoor tanning, sunless tanning, and sun protection behaviors do not seem to differ between sexual minority and heterosexual women.[46]

Smoking and Alcohol Use

Sexual minorities are more likely to report smoking, alcohol, substance use, and substance use disorders.[47] In a US population-based study, gay men reported a significantly lower prevalence of not currently smoking cigarettes (77.0% vs 81.4%) and moderate/no drinking (51.8% vs 60.8%) than heterosexual men. Similarly, lesbian women were significantly less likely than heterosexual women to report not currently smoking (66.2% vs 86.0%) and moderate/no drinking (50.6% vs 75.0%), respectively.[48] These findings concur with prior studies that gay males and gay/lesbian females are more likely to be current smokers than heterosexual males (25.3% vs 18.9%) and heterosexual females (23.8% vs 14.5%), respectively. Binge drinking is also significantly more common in bisexual males and females than their heterosexual counterparts (53.8% vs 39.6% for males; 35.3% vs 23.1% for females) but not in gay/lesbian individuals.[49]

Tobacco and alcohol use among sexual minorities may contribute to an increased risk of skin cancer. Tobacco use has been well-established to cause lung, bladder, and head and neck SCC. Limited evidence supports that smoking is associated with an increased risk of developing cSCC and possibly BCC.[50,51] A Dutch case-control study found that the relative risk (RR) for developing cSCC was 2-fold higher in smokers than nonsmokers ($P = .008$) with a significant dose–response relationship with the number of cigarettes and pipes smoked.[51] A meta-analysis using

US data found that female ever smokers compared with nonsmokers had a higher risk of cSCC (RR, 1.19; $P<.05$) and BCC (RR, 1.06; $P<.05$).[50] It is possible that higher rates of tobacco use among sexual minorities may increase their RR of keratinocytes carcinomas in comparison with heterosexuals.[50,52]

Alcohol use has also been associated with risk of keratinocyte carcinomas.[53,54] A systematic review and meta-analysis found that for every 0.35 ounce increase in ethanol intake per day, the risk of BCC and cSCC increased by 7% and 11%, respectively; this review included studies that controlled for UVR exposure.[55] Another systematic review and meta-analysis found an elevated RR for cutaneous melanoma in moderate-to-heavy drinkers, although this risk became statistically insignificant after adjusting for UVR exposure.[56] Increased rates of both alcohol and tobacco use thus may contribute to an increased risk of keratinocyte carcinomas and melanoma among sexual minorities.

Human Immunodeficiency Virus Infection

Sexual minorities—especially men who have sex with men (MSM)—are disproportionately impacted by sexual transmitted infections, including human immunodeficiency virus (HIV) infection. In 2017, 25,748 sexual minority men were diagnosed with HIV in the United States, accounting for 66% of all HIV diagnoses and 82% of diagnoses among men. Racial/ethnic and sexual minority men, moreover, face a particularly high burden of HIV. From 2012 to 2016, rates of HIV diagnoses increased 12% in Hispanic sexual minority men, and black sexual minority men continued to represent the largest absolute number of HIV diagnoses.[57] HIV infection in women who have sex with women is reported less frequently and remains difficult to establish accurately.[58] However, sexual minority women may engage in other high-risk behaviors (eg, injection drug use) and/or experience other health care disparities that place them at risk for HIV infection.[59]

Existing evidence supports that patients with HIV have an increased risk of developing cSCC.[60] A recent retrospective Danish cohort study found a 5.4-fold increased risk of cSCC in HIV-infected individuals compared with age- and sex-matched HIV-negative controls. The increased risk of cSCC correlated with immunosuppression status and was consistent regardless of HIV infection route. A similar study in a California-based population found that patients with HIV had a 2.6-fold increased risk of cSCC that was associated with lower CD4 counts and higher viral loads.[61,62] Given the potential viral-related pathogenesis of cSCC, it is biologically plausible that patients with poorly controlled HIV (ie, lower CD4 counts and high viral loads) are at an increased risk for cSCC, either through failure of tumor immune surveillance or through a potential oncovirus. Thus, increased rates of HIV among sexual minorities may contribute to an increased risk of cSCC.

These studies also identified an approximately 2-fold increased risk of BCC in patients with HIV.[60,61] In the Danish cohort study, this relationship was restricted to HIV-infected MSM and did not correlate with immunosuppression status.[60] In the California cohort study, HIV-infected MSM maintained the highest increased risk of BCC, whereas HIV-infected women demonstrated no increased RR of BCC, and no association was identified between BCC risk and immunosuppression.[61,62] These studies did not control for rates of UVR exposure behaviors such as tanning or sun protection behaviors. As the increased risk of BCC in HIV-infected individuals seems to be restricted to MSM and unrelated to immunosuppression, it is likely that differences in behavioral risk factors (such as UVR exposure), rather than immunosuppression, may better explain the higher rates of BCC found in HIV-infected persons.[63]

Human Papillomavirus Infection

Sexual minority men and women have an increased risk of human papillomavirus (HPV) infection.[64] In a systematic review and meta-analysis of HPV prevalence in China, 59.9% of MSM had at least 1 type of HPV. Strikingly, MSM demonstrated a significantly greater odds of infection with HPV compared with heterosexual men (59.0% vs 14.5%; OR, 8.81; $P<.05$). Overall, HIV-positive MSM had the highest prevalence of HPV (87.5%) among all patient populations.[65] The increased risk of HPV infection among MSM may be explained by higher rates of HIV infection and the higher number of lifetime sexual partners in these populations.[66] Sexual minority youth also report low compliance with HPV vaccination, which may predispose to HPV infection.[67,68]

Sexual minority women also have a significantly greater odds of infection with any HPV type (49.7% vs 41.1%; OR, 1.44; $P = .001$) and with a high-risk HPV type (37% vs 27.9%; OR, 1.52; $P<.001$) when compared with heterosexual women. Among all sexual minority women, bisexual women were more likely to have any HPV type (57.7% vs 35.5%) and a high-risk HPV type (43.6% vs 26.7%) than lesbians.[64] This increased risk of HPV may be due to a higher number of sexual partners in sexual minority women compared with heterosexual women, in addition to the paucity of sexual health education and programs directed at sexual minority women.[69]

High rates of HPV infection in sexual minorities may contribute to an increased risk of cSCC. Although oncogenic/high-risk HPV types (eg, HPV16, 18, 31, 33, 35, and 45) are the cause of almost all cervical cancers, these viruses also contribute to SCC of the penis, vulva, vagina, anus, oropharynx, and possibly cSCC.[70,71] Globally, almost 90% and 30% of anal and oropharyngeal SCCs, respectively, are attributable to HPV infection.[70] In the United States, up to 70% of oropharyngeal SCCs are thought to be secondary to HPV infection. SCC of the oropharynx continues to increase in incidence and is projected to become the most common HPV-related cancer.[72,73]

The role of HPV in cSCC is less established. Based on a systematic review and meta-analysis, cSCC were more likely to carry HPV than normal skin (pooled effect size, 3.43; $P<.0001$). Additionally, cSCC from immunosuppressed patients were more likely to carry HPV than cSCC from immunocompetent patients. Although this meta-analysis was limited by the heterogeneity of included studies, it does support an association between HPV and cSCC.[71] Further research is necessary to understand the relationship between HPV and cSCC, but current evidence suggests that increased rates of HPV in sexual minorities may contribute to an increased risk of skin cancer, particularly cSCC, among sexual minorities.

GENDER MINORITIES

There is less robust evidence on the burden of skin cancer and skin cancer risk factors in gender minorities. Much of the existing literature is largely limited to case reports specifically detailing the development of SCC in the neovagina of transwomen after gender affirmation surgery.[74,75] Although the risk of keratinocyte carcinomas and melanoma in gender minorities compared with cisgender persons is unknown, a number of risk factors are relevant to skin cancer among gender minorities.

Indoor Tanning

Indoor tanning behaviors among gender minorities are not well-studied. However, a recent study of Canadian adolescents demonstrated a higher prevalence of indoor tanning among gender minority youth.[76] Among male youth, persons identifying as transgender or another gender minority had a significantly higher odds of indoor tanning within their lifetime when compared with cisgender peers (12.9% vs 3.8%; OR, 2.75; $P<.001$). Of note, male youth identifying as trans or with another gender minority identity had higher rates of indoor tanning than sexual minority males (9.9%). Female youth identifying as trans or with another gender minority identity demonstrated a significantly higher odds of indoor tanning compared with cisgender females (12.6% vs 10.3%; OR, 1.41; P = .044).[76] Specific motivations for indoor tanning and rates of other tanning and sun protection behaviors have not been studied among gender minorities.

Smoking and Alcohol Use

Gender minority individuals also experience increased stress related to their minority status, contributing to higher rates of alcohol and tobacco use.[77,78] Alcohol use is highly prevalent among gender minority populations.[79] In a sample of 1210 transgender adults living in the United States, 21.5% of participants reported excessive alcohol use and this was correlated with their degree of gender dysphoria.[80] Gender minorities are also more likely to use tobacco than cisgender people.[81] In a cross-sectional survey of 174 transgender and 2372 cisgender adults, transgender compared with cisgender adults had a greater odds of being a current smoker (15.0% vs 9.0%; OR, 1.25) although this trend did not reach statistical significance.[81] As discussed, high rates of alcohol and tobacco use may contribute to an increased risk of keratinocyte carcinomas and melanoma in gender minorities.[50,53,54]

Human Immunodeficiency Virus Infection

HIV infection may also contribute to a higher risk of cSCC among gender minorities. An estimated 27.7% and 11.8% of transwomen and transmen, respectively, are currently infected with HIV in the United States.[82] HIV prevalence is 34 times higher in reproductive-age transwomen compared with cisgender women.[83] Racial/ethnic gender minorities demonstrate an even greater burden, as 56.3% of black transwomen are HIV positive.[82] Furthermore, previous studies have reported that HIV-positive gender minorities are less likely than cisgender HIV-positive patients to adhere to antiretroviral treatment and more likely to have lower CD4 counts and detectable viral loads.[84] The high burden of HIV among gender minorities may contribute to an increased risk of cSCC in gender minorities, especially among those with poorly controlled HIV.

Human Papillomavirus Infection

Gender minorities also have higher rates of HPV infection, which may contribute to an increased risk of cSCC.[85] In a prospective cohort study of 68 Peruvian transwomen, 95.6% had at least 1 anogenital HPV genotype and 19.1% had visible anogenital condyloma at baseline.[86] In an Italian study, 40% of transgender minority patients had detectable HPV DNA from anal, vaginal, and/or penile samples. More specifically, HPV DNA was found in 21.4% of transmen and 52.4% of transwomen. High risk subtypes were found in 93% of HPV-positive transgender individuals.[87] In a retrospective review of cytologic findings of neovaginas, 90% of samples had cytologically atypical features.[88]

Given the high burden of oncogenic HPV among gender minorities, especially among transwomen, there is a serious concern for HPV-related SCC.[74,85,89] In vaginoplasty, skin from the scrotum, penile shaft, or a combination of both are used as the donor graft or flap to construct the neovagina. These tissues are often at high risk of HPV infection before surgery and may be more susceptible to development of secondary malignancies owing to tissue damage and scarring from surgery. For instance, a case report of a 78-year-old transwoman demonstrated HPV-associated SCC in the neovagina constructed from penile and scrotal skin 45 years after vaginoplasty.[75] Although there is a plausible and demonstrated risk of SCC of the neovagina, the prevalence of SCC in neovaginas of transwomen who have undergone vaginoplasty is currently unknown.

Estrogen Therapy

Transwomen and other gender minority patients receiving feminizing hormone therapy with estrogen derivatives may be at a theoretic increased risk for melanoma. Although controversial, there are conflicting data demonstrating an association between estrogen exposure and melanoma. From a pathophysiology perspective, dysplastic nevi with severe cytologic atypia and lentigo maligna express estrogen receptors and may respond to estrogen stimulation.[90] A Norwegian cohort study of 684,696 women found that use of estrogen hormone replacement therapy was associated with an increased risk of melanoma (RR, 1.19) for both oral estrogen therapy (RR, 1.45) and vaginal estrogen therapy (RR, 1.44), but not for combination estrogen and progestin therapy (RR, 0.91).[91] A meta-analysis of 16,787 melanoma cases did not find any association between melanoma and use of oral contraceptives or hormone replacement therapy, although melanoma was positively associated with late age at first birth and negatively associated with multiparity, which are both associated with increased lifetime estrogen exposure.[92] In comparison, a French prospective study of 460 melanoma cases did not find an association between age at first birth and risk of melanoma. However, the risk of melanoma was decreased in women who were at least 15 years old at menarche (RR, 0.67) and younger than 48 years old at menopause (RR, 0.70) and women who reported irregular menstrual cycles (RR, 0.52) and shorter ovulatory life (RR, 0.52). These results support an increased risk of melanoma in association with estrogen exposure.[93] No study has yet investigated whether feminizing hormone therapy with estradiol is associated with an increased risk of skin cancer specifically among gender minorities receiving feminizing hormone therapy.[89] However, because gender minorities may experience a greater length of estrogen exposure in comparison with cisgender women on hormone replacement therapy, further investigation is needed.

FUTURE DIRECTIONS

SGM have unique risk factors and behaviors that may contribute to a differential risk of skin cancer. These include, but are not limited to, a high prevalence of indoor tanning and other risky tanning behaviors among sexual minority men, and increased rates of smoking, alcohol use, and HIV and HPV infection among SGM. Furthermore, transwomen and other gender minorities receiving feminizing hormone therapy with estrogen may have an increased risk for developing melanoma. It is therefore essential that we prioritize dermatologic research in SGM to improve our understanding of both the prevalence and potential risk factors for skin cancer in these populations. Such information will inform appropriate screening practices and contribute to the design of tailored interventions to reduce preventable behaviors that contribute to skin cancer disparities experienced by SGM.

DISCLOSURE

The authors have no commercial or financial conflicts of interest to disclose. The authors have no funding sources to disclose.

REFERENCES

1. Guy GP, Machlin SR, Ekwueme DU, et al. Prevalence and costs of skin cancer treatment in the U.S., 2002-2006 and 2007-2011. Am J Prev Med 2015;48(2):183–7.
2. Stern RS. Prevalence of a history of skin cancer in 2007: results of an incidence-based model. Arch Dermatol 2010;146(3):279–82.
3. Robinson JK. Sun exposure, sun protection, and vitamin D. JAMA 2005;294(12):1541–3.
4. Muzic JG, Schmitt AR, Wright AC, et al. Incidence and trends of basal cell carcinoma and cutaneous squamous cell carcinoma: a population-based study in Olmsted County, Minnesota, 2000 to 2010. Mayo Clin Proc 2017;92(6):890–8.
5. Skin cancer: incidence rate. American Academy of Dermatology. 2018. Available at. https://www.aad. org/media/stats/conditions/skin-cancer. Accessed January 14, 2019.
6. U.S. Department of Health and Human Services. The surgeon general's call to action to prevent skin cancer. Washington, DC: Dept of Health and Human Services, Office of the Surgeon General; 2014.
7. Gandini S, Sera F, Cattaruzza MS, et al. Meta-analysis of risk factors for cutaneous melanoma: II. Sun exposure. Eur J Cancer 2005;41(1):45–60.
8. Parkin DM, Mesher D, Sasieni P. 13. Cancers attributable to solar (ultraviolet) radiation exposure in the UK in 2010. Br J Cancer 2011;105(Suppl 2):S66–9.
9. Sexual & gender minority research office annual report. National Institutes of Health: Sexual and Gender Minority Research Office. 2017. Available at: https://dpcpsi.nih.gov/sites/default/files/FY2017_SG MRO_AnnualReport_RF508_FINAL_508.pdf. Accessed September 17, 2018.
10. Mayer KH, Bradford JB, Makadon HJ, et al. Sexual and gender minority health: what we know and what needs to be done. Am J Public Health 2008; 98(6):989–95.
11. Deutsch M. Guidelines for the primary and gender-affirming care of transgender and gender nonbinary people: introduction to the guidelines. Center of Excellence for Transgender Health. 2016. Available at: http://transhealth.ucsf.edu/pdf/ Transgender-PGACG-6-17-16.pdf. Accessed September 17, 2018.
12. Mansh M, Katz KA, Linos E, et al. Association of skin cancer and indoor tanning in sexual minority men and women. JAMA Dermatol 2015;151(12):1308–16.
13. Modenese A, Korpinen L, Gobba F. Solar radiation exposure and outdoor work: an underestimated occupational risk. Int J Environ Res Public Health 2018;15(10). https://doi.org/10.3390/ijerph15102063.
14. El Ghissassi F, Baan R, Straif K, et al. A review of human carcinogens—part D: radiation. Lancet Oncol 2009;10(8):751–2.
15. International Agency for Research on Cancer Working Group on artificial ultraviolet (UV) light and skin cancer. The association of use of sunbeds with cutaneous malignant melanoma and other skin cancers:

a systematic review. Int J Cancer 2007;120(5): 1116–22.

16. Wehner MR, Shive ML, Chren M-M, et al. Indoor tanning and non-melanoma skin cancer: systematic review and meta-analysis. BMJ 2012;345:e5909.

17. O'Sullivan DE, Brenner DR, Demers PA, et al. Indoor tanning and skin cancer in Canada: a meta-analysis and attributable burden estimation. Cancer Epidemiol 2019;59:1–7.

18. Lazovich D, Vogel RI, Berwick M, et al. Indoor tanning and risk of melanoma: a case-control study in a highly exposed population. Cancer Epidemiol Biomarkers Prev 2010;19(6):1557–68.

19. Guy GP, Berkowitz Z, Watson M, et al. Indoor tanning among young non-hispanic white females. JAMA Intern Med 2013;173(20):1920–2.

20. Guy GP, Berkowitz Z, Holman DM, et al. Recent changes in the prevalence of and factors associated with frequency of indoor tanning among US adults. JAMA Dermatol 2015;151(11):1256–9.

21. Mays D, Atkins MB, Ahn J, et al. Indoor tanning dependence in young adult women. Cancer Epidemiol Biomarkers Prev 2017;26(11):1636–43.

22. Myrick JG, Noar SM, Sontag JM, et al. Connections between sources of health and beauty information and indoor tanning behavior among college women. J Am Coll Health 2018;1–6. https://doi.org/10.1080/07448481.2018.1536662.

23. Gillen MM, Markey CN. The role of body image and depression in tanning behaviors and attitudes. Behav Med 2012;38(3):74–82.

24. Joel Hillhouse GC, Thompson JK, Jacobsen PB, et al. Investigating the role of appearance-based factors in predicting sunbathing and tanning salon use. J Behav Med 2009;32(6):532–44.

25. Frederick DA, Essayli J. Male body image: the roles of sexual orientation and body mass index across five national U.S. studies. Psychol Men Masc 2016; 17(4):336–51.

26. Griffiths S, Murray SB, Krug I, et al. The contribution of social media to body dissatisfaction, eating disorder symptoms, and anabolic steroid use among sexual minority men. Cyberpsychol Behav Soc Netw 2018;21(3):149–56.

27. Feldman MB, Meyer IH. Eating disorders in diverse lesbian, gay, and bisexual populations. Int J Eat Disord 2007;40(3):218–26.

28. Boroughs MS, Krawczyk R, Thompson JK. Body dysmorphic disorder among diverse racial/ethnic and sexual orientation groups: prevalence estimates and associated factors. Sex Roles 2010;63(9–10): 725–37.

29. Morrison MA, Morrison TG, Sager C-L. Does body satisfaction differ between gay men and lesbian women and heterosexual men and women? A meta-analytic review. Body Image 2004;1(2): 127–38.

30. Yeung H, Chen SC. Sexual orientation and indoor tanning device use: a population-based study. JAMA Dermatol 2016;152(1):99–101.

31. Blashill AJ. Indoor tanning and skin cancer risk among diverse US youth: results from a national sample. JAMA Dermatol 2017;153(3):344–5.

32. Blashill AJ, Safren SA. Skin cancer risk behaviors among US men: the role of sexual orientation. Am J Public Health 2014;104(9):1640–1.

33. Aubert PM, Seibyl JP, Price JL, et al. Dopamine efflux in response to ultraviolet radiation in addicted sunbed users. Psychiatry Res Neuroimaging 2016; 251:7–14.

34. Klimek P, Lamb KM, Nogg KA, et al. Current and ideal skin tone: associations with tanning behavior among sexual minority men. Body Image 2018;25:31–4.

35. Admassu N, Pimentel MA, Halley MC, et al. Motivations among sexual-minority men for starting and stopping indoor tanning. Br J Dermatol 2019. https://doi.org/10.1111/bjd.17684.

36. Blashill AJ, Pagoto S. Skin cancer risk in gay and bisexual men: a call to action. JAMA Dermatol 2015;151(12):1293–4.

37. Blashill AJ, Rooney BM, Wells KJ. An integrated model of skin cancer risk in sexual minority males. J Behav Med 2018;41(1):99–108.

38. Feldman SR, Liguori A, Kucenic M, et al. Ultraviolet exposure is a reinforcing stimulus in frequent indoor tanners. J Am Acad Dermatol 2004;51(1):45–51.

39. Zeller S, Lazovich D, Forster J, et al. Do adolescent indoor tanners exhibit dependency? J Am Acad Dermatol 2006;54(4):589–96.

40. Meyer IH. Prejudice, social stress, and mental health in lesbian, gay, and bisexual populations: conceptual issues and research evidence. Psychol Bull 2003;129(5):674–97.

41. Hatzenbuehler ML. How does sexual minority stigma "get under the skin"? A psychological mediation framework. Psychol Bull 2009;135(5):707–30.

42. Mosher CE, Danoff-Burg S. Addiction to indoor tanning: relation to anxiety, depression, and substance use. Arch Dermatol 2010;146(4):412–7.

43. Gao Y, Arron ST, Linos E, et al. Indoor tanning, sunless tanning, and sun-protection behaviors among sexual minority Men. JAMA Dermatol 2018;154(4): 477–9.

44. Dodds M, Arron ST, Linos E, et al. Characteristics and skin cancer risk behaviors of adult sunless tanners in the United States. JAMA Dermatol 2018; 154(9):1066–71.

45. Autier P, Boniol M, Doré J-F. Sunscreen use and increased duration of intentional sun exposure: still a burning issue. Int J Cancer 2007;121(1):1–5.

46. Yeung H, Baranowski MLH, Chen SC. Skin cancer risk factors and screening among sexual minority and heterosexual women. J Am Acad Dermatol 2019. https://doi.org/10.1016/j.jaad.2019.02.024.

47. Slater ME, Godette D, Huang B, et al. Sexual orientation-based discrimination, excessive alcohol use, and substance use disorders among sexual minority adults. LGBT Health 2017;4(5):337–44.

48. Cunningham TJ, Xu F, Town M. Prevalence of five health-related behaviors for chronic disease prevention among sexual and gender minority adults — 25 U.S. States and Guam, 2016. Morb Mortal Wkly Rep 2018;67(32):888–93.

49. Lunn MR, Cui W, Zack MM, et al. Sociodemographic characteristics and health outcomes among lesbian, gay, and bisexual U.S. adults using healthy people 2020 leading health indicators. LGBT Health 2017; 4(4):283–94.

50. Song F, Qureshi AA, Gao X, et al. Smoking and risk of skin cancer: a prospective analysis and a meta-analysis. Int J Epidemiol 2012;41(6):1694–705.

51. De Hertog SA, Wensveen CA, Bastiaens MT, et al. Relation between smoking and skin cancer. J Clin Oncol 2001;19(1):231–8.

52. Panelos J, Massi D. Emerging role of Notch signaling in epidermal differentiation and skin cancer. Cancer Biol Ther 2009;8(21):1986–93.

53. Wu S, Li W-Q, Qureshi AA, et al. Alcohol consumption and risk of cutaneous basal cell carcinoma in women and men: 3 prospective cohort studies. Am J Clin Nutr 2015;102(5):1158–66.

54. Siiskonen S, Han J, Li T, et al. Alcohol intake is associated with increased risk of squamous cell carcinoma of the skin: three US prospective cohort studies. Nutr Cancer 2016;68(4):545–53.

55. Yen H, Dhana A, Okhovat J-P, et al. Alcohol intake and risk of nonmelanoma skin cancer: a systematic review and dose-response meta-analysis. Br J Dermatol 2017;177(3):696–707.

56. Rota M, Pasquali E, Bellocco R, et al. Alcohol drinking and cutaneous melanoma risk: a systematic review and dose-risk meta-analysis. Br J Dermatol 2014;170(5):1021–8.

57. HIV in the United States and Dependent Areas. Centers for Disease Control and Prevention. 2019. Available at: https://www.cdc.gov/hiv/statistics/overview/ataglance.html. Accessed September 17, 2018.

58. Chan SK, Thornton LR, Chronister KJ, et al. Morbidity and mortality weekly report (MMWR): likely female-to-female sexual transmission of HIV — Texas, 2012. Centers for Disease Control and Prevention; 2014. p. 209–12.

59. HIV risk for lesbians, bisexuals & other women who have sex with women. Women's Institute at Gay Men's Health Crisis. 2009. Available at: http://www.gmhc.org/files/editor/file/GMHC_lap_whitepaper_0609.pdf. Accessed September 17, 2018.

60. Omland SH, Ahlström MG, Gerstoft J, et al. Risk of skin cancer in patients with HIV: a Danish nationwide cohort study. J Am Acad Dermatol 2018;79(4):689–95.

61. Silverberg MJ, Leyden W, Warton EM, et al. HIV infection status, immunodeficiency, and the incidence of non-melanoma skin cancer. J Natl Cancer Inst 2013;105(5):350–60.

62. Asgari MM, Ray GT, Quesenberry CP, et al. Association of multiple primary skin cancers with human immunodeficiency virus infection, CD4 count, and viral load. JAMA Dermatol 2017;153(9):892–6.

63. Mansh MD, Marks DH. Reply to: "Risk of skin cancer in HIV-infected patients: a Danish nationwide cohort study. J Am Acad Dermatol 2018. https://doi.org/10.1016/j.jaad.2018.07.067.

64. Reiter PL, McRee A-L. HPV infection among a population-based sample of sexual minority women from USA. Sex Transm Infect 2017;93(1):25–31.

65. Ma X, Wang Q, Ong JJ, et al. Prevalence of human papillomavirus by geographical regions, sexual orientation and HIV status in China: a systematic review and meta-analysis. Sex Transm Infect 2018; 94(6):434–42.

66. Meites E, Gorbach PM, Gratzer B, et al. Monitoring for human papillomavirus vaccine impact among gay, bisexual, and other men who have sex with men—United States, 2012–2014. J Infect Dis 2016; 214(5):689–96.

67. Reiter PL, McRee A-I, Katz ML, et al. Human papillomavirus vaccination among young adult gay and bisexual men in the United States. Am J Public Health 2015;105(1):96–102.

68. McRee A-L, Katz ML, Paskett ED, et al. HPV vaccination among lesbian and bisexual women: findings from a national survey of young adults. Vaccine 2014;32(37):4736–42.

69. Charlton BM, Reisner SL, Agénor M, et al. Sexual orientation disparities in human papillomavirus vaccination in a longitudinal cohort of U.S. males and females. LGBT Health 2017;4(3):202–9.

70. de Martel C, Plummer M, Vignat J, et al. Worldwide burden of cancer attributable to HPV by site, country and HPV type. Int J Cancer 2017;141(4):664–70.

71. Wang J, Aldabagh B, Yu J, et al. Role of human papillomavirus in cutaneous squamous cell carcinoma: a meta-analysis. J Am Acad Dermatol 2014; 70(4):621–9.

72. Pytynia KB, Dahlstrom KR, Sturgis EM. Epidemiology of HPV-associated oropharyngeal cancer. Oral Oncol 2014;50(5):380–6.

73. HPV and Oropharyngeal Cancer. Centers for Disease Control and Prevention. 2018. Available at: https://www.cdc.gov/cancer/hpv/basic_info/hpv_oropharyngeal.htm. Accessed September 17, 2018.

74. Harder Y, Erni D, Banic A. Squamous cell carcinoma of the penile skin in a neovagina 20 years after male-to-female reassignment. Br J Plast Surg 2002;55(5):449–51.

75. Bollo J, Balla A, Rodriguez Luppi C, et al. HPV-related squamous cell carcinoma in a neovagina

after male-to-female gender confirmation surgery. Int J STD AIDS 2018;29(3):306–8.

76. Harland E, Griffith J, Lu H, et al. Health behaviours associated with indoor tanning based on the 2012/13 Manitoba Youth Health Survey. Health Promot Chronic Dis Prev Can 2016;36(8):149–62.

77. Coulter RWS, Blosnich JR, Bukowski LA, et al. Differences in alcohol use and alcohol-related problems between transgender- and nontransgender-identified young adults. Drug Alcohol Depend 2015;154:251–9.

78. Gamarel KE, Mereish EH, Manning D, et al. Minority stress, smoking patterns, and cessation attempts: findings from a community-sample of transgender women in the San Francisco Bay area. Nicotine Tob Res 2016;18(3):306–13.

79. Gilbert PA, Pass LE, Keuroghlian AS, et al. Alcohol research with transgender populations: a systematic review and recommendations to strengthen future studies. Drug Alcohol Depend 2018;186:138–46.

80. Gonzalez CA, Gallego JD, Bockting WO. Demographic characteristics, components of sexuality and gender, and minority stress and their associations to excessive alcohol, cannabis, and illicit (Non-cannabis) drug use among a large sample of transgender people in the United States. J Prim Prev 2017;38(4):419–45.

81. Fredriksen-Goldsen KI, Cook-Daniels L, Kim H-J, et al. Physical and mental health of transgender older adults: an at-risk and underserved population. Gerontologist 2014;54(3):488–500.

82. Herbst JH, Jacobs ED, Finlayson TJ, et al. Estimating HIV prevalence and risk behaviors of transgender persons in the United States: a systematic review. AIDS Behav 2008;12(1):1–17.

83. Clark H, Babu AS, Wiewel EW, et al. Diagnosed HIV Infection in transgender adults and adolescents: results from the National HIV Surveillance System, 2009–2014. AIDS Behav 2017;21(9):2774–83.

84. Xia Q, Seyoum S, Wiewel EW, et al. Reduction in gaps in high cd4 count and viral suppression

between transgender and cisgender persons living with HIV in New York City, 2007-2016. Am J Public Health 2018;e1–6. https://doi.org/10.2105/AJPH.2018.304748.

85. Brown B, Poteat T, Marg L, et al. Human papillomavirus-related cancer surveillance, prevention, and screening among transgender men and women: neglected populations at high risk. LGBT Health 2017;4(5):315–9.

86. Brown B, Galea JT, Byraiah G, et al. Anogenital human papillomavirus infection and HIV infection outcomes among Peruvian transgender women: results from a cohort study. Transgend Health 2016;1(1):94–8.

87. Loverro G, Di Naro E, Caringella AM, et al. Prevalence of human papillomavirus infection in a clinic sample of transsexuals in Italy. Sex Transm Infect 2016;92(1):67–9.

88. Grosse A, Grosse C, Lenggenhager D, et al. Cytology of the neovagina in transgender women and individuals with congenital or acquired absence of a natural vagina. Cytopathology 2017;28(3):184–91.

89. Mundluru SN, Larson AR. Medical dermatologic conditions in transgender women. Int J Womens Dermatol 2018;4(4):212–5.

90. Schmidt AN, Nanney LB, Boyd AS, et al. Oestrogen receptor-beta expression in melanocytic lesions. Exp Dermatol 2006;15(12):971–80.

91. Botteri E, Støer NC, Sakshaug S, et al. Menopausal hormone therapy and risk of melanoma: do estrogens and progestins have a different role? Int J Cancer 2017;141(9):1763–70.

92. Gandini S, Iodice S, Koomen E, et al. Hormonal and reproductive factors in relation to melanoma in women: current review and meta-analysis. Eur J Cancer 2011;47(17):2607–17.

93. Kvaskoff M, Bijon A, Mesrine S, et al. Cutaneous melanoma and endogenous hormonal factors: a large French prospective study. Am J Epidemiol 2011;173(10):1192–202.

Acne and the Lesbian, Gay, Bisexual, or Transgender Teenager

Laura Ragmanauskaite, BS, Benjamin Kahn, MD, BaoChau Ly, BS, Howa Yeung, MD, MSc*

KEYWORDS

- Acne • Dermatology • Lesbian • Gay • Bisexual • Transgender • Sexual and gender minority
- Isotretinoin

KEY POINTS

- Comprehensive care for moderate to severe acne in sexual and gender minority adolescents should include culturally competent discussions of sexual health, contraception, and/or gender-affirming therapy.
- Dermatologists should consider psychosocial factors and mental health issues, such as depression and suicidal ideation, in sexual and gender minority teenagers with acne.
- Gender-affirming hormone therapies in transgender and gender nonbinary teenagers impact acne presentation, treatment, and prognosis.

INTRODUCTION

Acne vulgaris affects approximately 85% of adolescents.[1] For sexual and gender minority (SGM) teenagers, management of acne could be more challenging. Despite multiple well-established clinical practice guidelines on acne management from the American Academy of Dermatology and the American Acne and Rosacea Society, there is little guidance on the specific best practices of acne care for SGM adolescent patients.[2,3] In this article, the authors review the current literature pertaining to comprehensive acne care for SGM adolescents. First, comprehensive care for moderate to severe acne in SGM adolescents should include culturally competent sexual health and contraceptive discussion.[4] Second, dermatologists should consider psychosocial factors and mental health issues, such as depression and suicidal ideation, in SGM teenagers with acne.[5,6] Last, gender-affirming hormone therapies in transgender and gender nonbinary teenagers specifically impact acne presentation, treatment, and prognosis.

DISCUSSIONS OF SEXUAL BEHAVIORS AND CONTRACEPTION IN ACNE CARE

SGM is an umbrella term encompassing "lesbian, gay, bisexual, and transgender populations as well as those whose sexual orientation, gender identity and expressions, or reproductive development varies from traditional, societal, cultural, or physiological norms."[7] Clinicians should become familiar with relevant terminology and health issues to become culturally competent with caring for SGM patients.[8–10] Using patient-preferred language, including names, pronouns, and any terms for their sexual orientation, gender identity, sexual behavior, or anatomy, is crucial in building therapeutic rapport.[8–10]

Cultural competency is especially important in the context of moderate to severe acne treatment. Selection of acne treatments in SGM patients

Department of Dermatology, Emory University School of Medicine, 1525 Clifton Road Northeast Suite 100, Atlanta, GA 30322, USA
* Corresponding author.
E-mail address: howa.yeung@emory.edu

Dermatol Clin 38 (2020) 219–226
https://doi.org/10.1016/j.det.2019.10.006
0733-8635/20/Published by Elsevier Inc.

largely follows the recommendations from current clinical practice guidelines.[2,3] In many cases of moderate to severe acne, oral medications, such as combination oral contraceptives, as well as teratogenic drugs, such as tetracyclines or isotretinoin, are required.[3] Specific consideration regarding sexual behaviors should be considered in all patients with reproductive potential, including postmenarchal SGM patients with functional female reproductive organs. Because sexual orientation and behaviors may be fluid, frank discussions of sexual behaviors, safer sex practices, and reliable contraception are crucial.

To set the stage for normalized discussions of sex, gender, and sexual health with both SGM and non-SGM adolescents, it is crucial for clinicians to have a working knowledge of the clinical and medicolegal aspects of consent and confidentiality in minors.[11,12] Adolescents, particularly those at high risk of unintended pregnancy such as SGM youth, often cite confidentiality concerns as the reason to forgo health care, let alone sexual health and contraceptive care.[13,14] Although the US Health Insurance Portability and Accountability Act (HIPAA) law allows parental access to the minor's health records, a minor can consent to confidential sexual health care under appropriate state laws or if the parent agrees that the minor may have confidential care.[15] Clinicians should become familiar with state-specific laws regarding contraceptive services. As of April 1, 2019, 21 states and the District of Columbia explicitly allow all minors to access contraception, whereas 25 states affirm minor consent under specific circumstances based on age, marital status, or pregnancy status.[16] Moreover, HIPAA law also allows the clinician to exercise professional judgment to deny parental access to a minor's protected health information.[12]

Confidentiality should be addressed with the adolescent and parents at the initial visit, because many teens are unaware of the availability of confidential care.[17] The American Academy of Pediatrics recommends clinicians have an office policy that explicitly describes available confidential services and to discuss and document confidentiality with all parents and adolescents.[12] Discussion of care, with the parents present as well as reviewing with the adolescent patient alone, is an important step to encourage honest discussions of sexual health and contraception as relevant to acne care. Studies have demonstrated that discussion of sensitive health topics has a positive impact on youth perceptions of care provided.[18] Creating a safe and comfortable environment is especially important for SGM youth, who also are subject to lack of health care access, advocacy, and physician advice.[19] Dermatologists must therefore take on the important role of patient educator and advocate, beyond just taking an appropriate sexual health history, counseling contraceptives, and providing contraceptive access.

Clinicians should also inquire about sexual orientation, gender identity, and sexual behaviors when treating patients with moderate to severe acne. Without specifically addressing these factors, clinicians may be unaware of their adolescent patients' SGM status, despite its clinical relevance to acne care. A patient's sexual history may be complicated and require further questioning for the purpose of better acne care and counseling. For example, a female adolescent identifying as a lesbian may have current sexual encounters with women only, but had prior sexual encounters with men. A second example is a masculine-presenting patient with severe acne who identifies as nonbinary, was assigned female sex at birth, and may be sexually active with both men and women. These scenarios would require different contraceptive discussions before starting potentially teratogenic acne medications.

Specific and unambiguous discussions about safe sex practices and contraception are required because of varying health literacy among adolescents.[20] Misconception of pregnancy potential and contraceptive efficacy among all adolescents is common.[21] In a survey of 2314 "millennial" Americans born between the years 1980 and 2000, 19% received sex education classes in high school only and not middle school, and 23% did not have any classes in middle or high school at all.[22] Only 12% received sex education inclusive of same-sex relationships.[22] In addition, prior studies suggested that adolescents who report practicing abstinence may actually engage in penis-vagina sexual intercourse on occasion.[23] Therefore, strict adherence implies that strict adherence to abstinence while taking isotretinoin may be difficult, particularly for those who have previously been sexually active. One study demonstrated that 19% of previously sexually active adult women, of whom 95% self-identified as heterosexual and chose abstinence as their primary contraception admitted to having sexual intercourse during isotretinoin treatment. Furthermore, 31% of women who selected 2 forms of contraception had sex at least once without using both forms of contraception.[24] Therefore, before starting oral treatments for moderate to severe acne in women, unless the patient has never been sexually active with men, discussion of contraception will be crucial to prevent potential teratogenicity.

Clinicians should also be aware that the normal development of sexual identity may vary among adolescents. For example, awareness of sexual attraction may begin around an average age of 9 to 10, whereas self-labeling as lesbian, gay, or bisexual may follow at an average of age 16.[7] In addition to age variance, acceptance and disclosure of same-sex orientation, gender identity, and first sexual experience may vary widely.[7] Widespread stigma and discrimination in health care settings may further complicate acceptance and disclosure ages for SGM youth.[8,25] Therefore, it is important for clinicians to create a welcoming and nonjudgmental environment that facilitates comprehensive acne care.

PSYCHOSOCIAL IMPACT OF ACNE IN SEXUAL AND GENDER MINORITY PATIENTS

Among teenagers, acne is associated with lower levels of self-esteem and higher levels of depression and suicidal ideation.[5] Acne may lead to withdrawal from social activities and relationships.[26] Acne may be associated with increased mental health–related hospitalizations and associated costs among patients with mental health diagnoses.[27]

The psychosocial effects of acne may be compounded in SGM patients, who have higher baseline risks of mental health issues compared with heterosexual peers.[28] A national cross-sectional study of 4094 heterosexual and 564 sexual minority young adults aged 18 to 28 years showed that acne and sexual minority status are both associated with depression and suicidal ideation. The reported odds of suicidal ideation within the past 12 months associated with acne is higher for sexual minorities (35.4% with acne vs 15.3% without acne), as compared with heterosexuals (7.8% with acne vs 5.3% without acne; P for interaction between acne and sexual minority status = 0.04).[6] Because the quality-of-life impact of acne often does not correlate with objective measures of acne severity, it is important for dermatologists to routinely inquire and address the negative psychosocial impact of acne in SGM teenagers.[29,30]

Dermatologists should incorporate discussion of mental health impact of acne for SGM teens taking isotretinoin for mental health issues, particularly in the context of isotretinoin treatment for severe, nodular, or recalcitrant acne.[28] Although the research linking isotretinoin and depression and suicidal ideation has been controversial, dermatologists should be vigilant in screening for depression, given that the SGM patient population is already at an increased risk for mental health comorbidities.[31–34] Although noting that a history

of mental health disorder is a relative contraindication for isotretinoin treatment, avoiding isotretinoin treatment summarily in this population deprives patients from effective treatment of acne and its negative effects on mental health. The Patient Health Questionnaire-9 (PHQ-9) has been used to screen for depression in both adult and adolescent patients. For adolescents aged 13 to 17 years, a PHQ-9 score of ≥ 11 has a sensitivity of 89.5% and a specificity of 77.5% for detecting major depression by Diagnostic and Statistical Manual of Mental Disorders (Fourth Edition) criteria.[35] The PHQ-9 has been advocated for use in screening for active depression and suicidal ideation at every visit before, during, and after isotretinoin treatment.[36] Recent meta-analyses have concluded isotretinoin treatment may improve symptoms of depression in patients with severe acne.[33,34] It may also unduly create disparities in acne care access in SGM youth. Instead, dermatologists can facilitate both acne and mental health care access by providing routine screening and expediting referral to mental health professionals.

ACNE IN THE CONTEXT OF GENDER-AFFIRMING TREATMENT

Gender dysphoria is defined as significant distress owing to the marked incongruence between someone's expressed or experienced gender (gender identity) and one's sex assigned at birth based on reproductive organs.[1,37] Transgender and gender nonbinary patients often suffer the effects of gender dysphoria and require gender-affirming treatments, which may include hormonal therapy. Dermatologists should understand gender-affirming therapies, such as "puberty blockers" and cross-sex hormone therapies, because they have important implications on acne treatment and prognosis.

Puberty Blockers

Endogenous pubertal development may trigger or worsen gender dysphoria in transgender and gender nonbinary youth.[1,29] Acne also occurs during the onset of puberty and may therefore worsen gender dysphoria. To prevent irreversible development of secondary sex characteristics and other phenotypic changes incongruent with an individual's gender identity, the Endocrine Society and the World Professional Association for Transgender Health recommend puberty hormone suppression, or "puberty blockers." These treatments include gonadotropin-releasing hormone agonists, such as leuprolide injection or subcutaneous histrelin.[38,39] Notably, gonadotropin-releasing hormone agonists have been used to treat acne and hirsutism in adult populations.[40] The use of puberty blockers in transgender teenagers has increased drastically with the average age of therapy initiation starting around 14 years old.[41] This trend will likely continue as insurance companies change their policies to be more inclusive of transgender medical needs.[42] As such, peripubertal adolescents with acne and gender dysphoria should be referred to pediatric endocrinologists for consideration of puberty suppression and a discussion of gender-affirming therapy, in addition to guideline-based treatment of acne.

Testosterone Therapy

Current guidelines recommend gender-affirming hormones, such as testosterone therapy, for adolescent patients with persistent gender dysphoria and the capacity to provide informed consent, usually by the age of 16.[39] Testosterone therapy is a common treatment of transgender men, or biological women who identify as men, that induces the development of secondary male sex characteristics. However, the Endocrine Society guidelines recommend that "clinicians evaluate and address medical conditions [such as acne] that can be exacerbated by hormone depletion and treatment with sex hormones of the affirmed gender before beginning treatment."[39]

It is well known that the pathogenesis of acne is multifactorial, involving hormonal regulation, hyperkeratinization, increased sebum production, *Propionibacterium acnes* colonization, genetics, and environmental factors.[43,44] 5α-Reductase and 17β-hydroxysteroid dehydrogenase work to balance testosterone and dihydrotestosterone (DHT) production within sebaceous glands.[45] Testosterone and DHT bind to androgen receptors on sebaceous cells, which increase sebaceous gland diameter and sebum production.[46] Increased activity of certain 5α-reductase isoforms is also associated with the increased keratinocyte hyperproliferation and formation of microcomedones. Androgens create excess keratinization and increased sebum production that favor acne development.[47]

As a result, transmasculine patients who start testosterone therapy often develop or have worsening acne.[8] Although there are limited data on the natural history of acne in adolescents, existing studies in adults provide some evidence showing that acne develops within 4 to 6 months of testosterone initiation and may continue to evolve within the first 2 years.[48] A prospective study of 20 transmasculine patients found both facial and back/chest acne increased in prevalence over the first 6 months of testosterone therapy, from 35% to 82% and 15% to 88%, respectively.[49] Of patients, 55% had facial acne and 50% had chest/back acne after 1 year of testosterone therapy. Acne symptoms were typically mild with only 20% classified as moderate. A cross-sectional study of 50 transgender men averaging 10 years of testosterone therapy found that 70% had persistent acne symptoms. A recent study of 55 transmasculine patients on ≥2 years of testosterone therapy found the incidence of new-onset acne to be 38%.[50] Incidence of acne was correlated with serum testosterone levels greater than 630 ng/dL.[50] Another prospective study of 17 transgender men beginning hormone therapy found that more than 50% developed facial and back acne after 4 months of treatment.[51] Back acne was more common and severe than facial acne. This pattern follows the typical acne distribution found among cisgender men.[52] Current guidelines suggest hormone providers should assess patients every 3 months for adverse effects, including acne.[53]

There is no evidence-based guideline on the best practices for treating hormonal acne in the context of testosterone therapy. Clinicians currently rely on the general guidelines developed for cisgender populations.[2,8] Some common acne treatments, such as hormone antagonists, may not be appropriate for transgender patients.[54] However, given the known effect of testosterone on comedo formation, topical and/or systemic retinoids are crucial in addressing the first step of acne development.

Isotretinoin Treatment Considerations

Although some patients on exogenous testosterone have improvement of their acne over the first 2 years, some develop severe, nodular, or recalcitrant acne that require oral isotretinoin.[55,56] Isotretinoin does not interfere with exogenous testosterone therapy but it does pose several unique challenges for transgender patients. Isotretinoin may be associated with delayed wound healing that persists for 6 to 12 months after its discontinuation.[57] Patients planning to undergo gender-affirming surgeries should be aware of this potential side effect because it could delay their transition or affect the aesthetic results from their surgery. Dermatologists considering isotretinoin should discuss the patient's goals and plans regarding any surgical procedures. In addition, although parental consent may be waived in the context of sexual health, parental consent is required for isotretinoin treatment in minors.[58,59]

The teratogenic side effects of isotretinoin create additional treatment considerations for transgender patients. Patients' sexual behaviors, gender identity, and history of gender-affirming therapy affect their risk for pregnancy and potential need for contraception. Some transmasculine patients may have had a hysterectomy and/or bilateral oophorectomy as part of gender-affirming surgical treatment and do not have the potential for pregnancy. On the other hand, a transmasculine person with a functional uterus and ovaries still has pregnancy potential if he engages in penis-vagina sexual intercourse with men, even if he were receiving testosterone therapy and were amenorrheic.[60] Such complicated sexual histories must be elicited for appropriate counseling and enrollment in the iPLEDGE program, as detailed in later discussion.

The Food and Drug Administration currently requires all patients initiating or receiving isotretinoin to participate in iPLEDGE, a registry aimed at preventing isotretinoin-exposed pregnancy.[32] When working with lesbian, gay, bisexual, transgender, and queer/questioning acne patients, clinicians must help select the appropriate contraceptive options within iPLEDGE, keeping in mind the patient's current or future sexual activity and reproductive potential. For instance, iPLEDGE allows female patients to select complete abstinence with men as a reliable contraceptive method. Transmasculine patients and cisgender lesbian patients who have reproductive potential, who are exclusively sexually active with cisgender women and do not have penis-vagina intercourse, may also select abstinence as a contraceptive method. Nevertheless, patients who cannot commit to complete abstinence from penis-vagina intercourse and have not undergone bottom surgeries (ie, phalloplasty and metoidioplasty) will require 2 forms of reliable contraception.[24]

For transmasculine patients interested in oral contraception, progestin-based long-acting reversible contraception is indicated and does not interfere with testosterone therapy.[61] Furthermore, intrauterine devices with progestins containing levonorgestrel, intradermal etonogestrel implants, or depot medroxyprogesterone acetate injections provide the additional gender-affirming benefits of decreased menstrual bleeding and/or induction of amenorrhea in transmasculine or nonbinary adolescents.[62] Progesterone-only pills or exogenous testosterone alone does not meet current iPLEDGE guidelines on contraception. Although combination oral contraceptive pills may be used, many patients prefer to avoid estrogens given potential concern about feminizing effects that may be counterproductive to their transition goals.[62] Multidisciplinary care with knowledgeable family planning providers will be essential to ensure appropriate provision of contraceptive care.

Dermatologists should also be aware that the language and pregnancy prevention guidelines in iPLEDGE were developed for cisgender women. iPLEDGE requires patients to gender-identify based on their sex at birth.[58,60,63] Transgender and gender nonbinary patients assigned female gender at birth are required to sign documentation that identifies them as "female patients who can get pregnant." Signing the iPledge may be psychologically traumatic because it asks patients to choose between treating their acne and affirming their gender identity, with some patients choosing to forgo acne treatment.[64] In the authors' experience, individualized discussion of ongoing advocacy efforts by dermatologists to promote gender-inclusive changes to the iPLEDGE system may help develop a therapeutic alliance, allay patient concerns regarding cultural competency of the provider, and facilitate access to isotretinoin treatment.[60,63,64]

Estrogen/Antiandrogen Therapy

For transfemale or nonbinary patients undergoing estrogen and/or antiandrogen therapy, acne may be improved by several potential mechanisms, including direct opposition of androgens, negative feedback loop on gonadotrophin release, and/or gene modulation responsible for sebum and lipid production.[65,66] Many transfeminine patients receiving estradiol and antiandrogens, such as spironolactone, often notice improvement in their acne.[43] For transfeminine patients with acne recalcitrant to hormone therapy, endocrine evaluation to titrate feminizing hormone doses and to rule out underlying hyperandrogenic states should be considered.

Other Considerations

Chest binding involves the use of ace bandages or elastic bands to tightly bind breasts in order to achieve a more masculine contour.[67,68] Although 1 small study suggested that chest binding does not negatively affect acne severity in transgender men receiving testosterone,[52] there have been reports of acne and folliculitis, along with itching, pain, and scarring, associated with prolonged chest-binding practices.[68] Cosmetics and make up is another means for patients to explore or affirm their gender identity or sexual identity. Discussion of cosmetic use and anticipatory guidance regarding noncomedogenic products should be provided.[69]

SUMMARY

Most adolescents experience acne vulgaris during puberty regardless of their sexual orientation or gender identity. For SGM adolescents, however, comprehensive acne care requires dermatologists to actively engage in culturally competent discussions of sexual health, contraception, and/or gender-affirming therapy. Dermatologists should recognize that acne and SGM status are both independent risk factors for mental health comorbidity, including depression and suicide. Screening and referral to mental health providers should accompany, rather than hinder, moderate to severe acne care for SGM adolescents who suffer from both acne and mental health disorders. Gender-affirming hormone therapy is associated with changes in acne presentation and severity. Dermatologists should help transgender or gender nonbinary adolescents navigate sexual health, contraceptive, and logistical considerations in accessing isotretinoin for the treatment of severe acne.

DISCLOSURE

Dr H. Yeung was supported in part by the National Center for Advancing Translational Sciences of the National Institutes of Health under award number UL1TR002378 and KL2TR002381. The content is solely the responsibility of the authors and does not necessarily represent the official views of the National Institutes of Health. Dr H. Yeung has received honorarium from Syneos (InVentiv) Health. All other authors disclosed no financial conflicts of interest.

REFERENCES

1. Lynn DD, Umari T, Dunnick CA, et al. The epidemiology of acne vulgaris in late adolescence. Adolesc Health Med Ther 2016;7:13–25.
2. Zaenglein AL, Pathy AL, Schlosser BJ, et al. Guidelines of care for the management of acne vulgaris. J Am Acad Dermatol 2016;74(5):945–73.e33.
3. Eichenfield LF, Krakowski AC, Piggott C, et al. Evidence-based recommendations for the diagnosis and treatment of pediatric acne. Pediatrics 2013; 131(Suppl 3):S163–86.
4. Marks DH, Awosika O, Rengifo-Pardo M, et al. Dermatologic surgical care for transgender individuals. Dermatol Surg 2019;45(3):446–57.
5. Halvorsen JA, Stern RS, Dalgard F, et al. Suicidal ideation, mental health problems, and social impairment are increased in adolescents with acne: a population-based study. J Invest Dermatol 2011; 131(2):363–70.
6. Gao Y, Wei EK, Arron ST, et al. Acne, sexual orientation, and mental health among young adults in the United States: a population-based, cross-sectional study. J Am Acad Dermatol 2017;77(5):971–3.
7. The Institute of Medicine Committee on Lesbian, Gay, Bisexual, and Transgender Health Issues and Research Gaps and Opportunities. The health of lesbian, gay, bisexual, and transgender people: building a foundation for better understanding. Washington, DC: Institute of Medicine; 2011.
8. Rafferty J, Committee on Psychosocial Aspects of Child and Family Health, Committee on Adolescence, Section on Lesbian, Gay, Bisexual, and Transgender Health and Wellness. Ensuring comprehensive care and support for transgender and gender-diverse children and adolescents. Pediatrics 2018;142(4) [pii:e20182162].
9. Yeung H, Luk KM, Chen SC, et al. Dermatologic care for lesbian, gay, bisexual, and transgender persons: epidemiology, screening, and disease prevention. J Am Acad Dermatol 2019;80(3):591–602.
10. Yeung H, Luk KM, Chen SC, et al. Dermatologic care for lesbian, gay, bisexual, and transgender persons: terminology, demographics, health disparities, and approaches to care. J Am Acad Dermatol 2019; 80(3):581–9.
11. The Joint Commission. Advancing effective communication, cultural competence and patient-and family-centered care for the lesbian, gay, bisexual and transgender (LGBT) community: a field guide. Oak Brook, IL: 2011.
12. Ott MA, Sucato GS, Committee on A. Contraception for adolescents. Pediatrics 2014;134(4):e1257–81.
13. Lehrer JA, Pantell R, Tebb K, et al. Forgone health care among U.S. adolescents: associations between risk characteristics and confidentiality concern. J Adolesc Health 2007;40(3):218–26.
14. Levine DA, Committee On Adolescence. Office-based care for lesbian, gay, bisexual, transgender, and questioning youth. Pediatrics 2013;132(1): e297–313.
15. Committee on Adolescence. Contraception for adolescents. Pediatrics 2014;134(4):e1244–56.
16. Guttmacher Institute. Minors' access to contraceptive services. 2019. Available at: https://www.guttmacher.org/state-policy/explore/minors-access-contraceptive-services. Accessed April 4, 2019.
17. Klein JD, McNulty M, Flatau CN. Adolescents' access to care: teenagers' self-reported use of services and perceived access to confidential care. Arch Pediatr Adolesc Med 1998;152(7):676–82.
18. Brown JD, Wissow LS. Discussion of sensitive health topics with youth during primary care visits: relationship to youth perceptions of care. J Adolesc Health 2009;44(1):48–54.
19. Luk JW, Gilman SE, Haynie DL, et al. Sexual orientation differences in adolescent health care access

and health-promoting physician advice. J Adolesc Health 2017;61(5):555–61.

20. Hubach RD. Disclosure matters: enhancing patient-provider communication is necessary to improve the health of sexual minority adolescents. J Adolesc Health 2017;61(5):537–8.

21. Chacko MR, Wiemann CM, Buzi RS, et al. Choice of postpartum contraception: factors predisposing pregnant adolescents to choose less effective methods over long-acting reversible contraception. J Adolesc Health 2016;58(6):628–35.

22. Jones RP, Cox D. How race and religion shape millenial attitudes on sexuality and reproductive health. Washington, DC: Public Religion Research Institute; 2015.

23. Bruckner H, Bearman P. After the promise: the STD consequences of adolescent virginity pledges. J Adolesc Health 2005;36(4):271–8.

24. Collins MK, Moreau JF, Opel D, et al. Compliance with pregnancy prevention measures during isotretinoin therapy. J Am Acad Dermatol 2014; 70(1):55–9.

25. Liszewski W, Peebles JK, Yeung H, et al. Persons of nonbinary gender–awareness, visibility, and health disparities. N Engl J Med 2018;379(25):2391–3.

26. Revol O, Milliez N, Gerard D. Psychological impact of acne on 21st-century adolescents: decoding for better care. Br J Dermatol 2015;172(Suppl 1):52–8.

27. Singam V, Rastogi S, Patel KR, et al. The mental health burden in acne vulgaris and rosacea: an analysis of the US National Inpatient Sample. Clin Exp Dermatol 2019;44(7):766–72.

28. Becerra-Culqui TA, Liu Y, Nash R, et al. Mental health of transgender and gender nonconforming youth compared with their peers. Pediatrics 2018; 141(5) [pii:e20173845].

29. Torjesen I. Managing acne female-to-male transgender persons. 2018. Available at: https://www.dermatologytimes.com/current-and-emerging-treatments-acne/managing-acne-female-male-transgender-persons. Accessed March 5, 2019.

30. Mallon E, Newton JN, Klassen A, et al. The quality of life in acne: a comparison with general medical conditions using generic questionnaires. Br J Dermatol 1999;140(4):672–6.

31. Marqueling AL, Zane LT. Depression and suicidal behavior in acne patients treated with isotretinoin: a systematic review. Semin Cutan Med Surg 2007; 26(4):210–20.

32. Oliveira JM, Sobreira G, Velosa J, et al. Association of isotretinoin with depression and suicide: a review of current literature. J Cutan Med Surg 2018;22(1): 58–64.

33. Li C, Chen J, Wang W, et al. Use of isotretinoin and risk of depression in patients with acne: a systematic review and meta-analysis. BMJ Open 2019;9(1): e021549.

34. Huang YC, Cheng YC. Isotretinoin treatment for acne and risk of depression: a systematic review and meta-analysis. J Am Acad Dermatol 2017; 76(6):1068–76.e9.

35. Richardson LP, McCauley E, Grossman DC, et al. Evaluation of the Patient Health Questionnaire-9 Item for detecting major depression among adolescents. Pediatrics 2010;126(6):1117–23.

36. Schrom K, Nagy T, Mostow E. Depression screening using health questionnaires in patients receiving oral isotretinoin for acne vulgaris. J Am Acad Dermatol 2016;75(1):237–9.

37. American Psychiatric Association. Diagnostic and Statistical Manual of Mental Disorders: Diagnostic and Statistical Manual of Mental Disorders. Fifth Edition. Arlington, VA: American Psychiatric Association; 2013.

38. Coleman E, Bockting W, Botzer M, et al. Standards of care for the health of transsexual, transgender, and gender-nonconforming people, version 7. Int J Transgend 2012;13(4):165–232.

39. Hembree WC, Cohen-Kettenis PT, Gooren L, et al. Endocrine treatment of gender-dysphoric/gender-incongruent persons: an Endocrine Society clinical practice guideline. J Clin Endocrinol Metab 2017; 102(11):3869–903.

40. Faloia E, Filipponi S, Mancini V, et al. Treatment with a gonadotropin-releasing hormone agonist in acne or idiopathic hirsutism. J Endocrinol Invest 1993; 16(9):675–7.

41. Lopez CM, Solomon D, Boulware SD, et al. Trends in the use of puberty blockers among transgender children in the United States. J Pediatr Endocrinol Metab 2018;31(6):665–70.

42. Stevens J, Gomez-Lobo V, Pine-Twaddell E. Insurance coverage of puberty blocker therapies for transgender youth. Pediatrics 2015;136(6): 1029–31.

43. Giltay EJ, Gooren LJ. Effects of sex steroid deprivation/administration on hair growth and skin sebum production in transsexual males and females. J Clin Endocrinol Metab 2000;85(8):2913–21.

44. Suh DH, Kwon HH. What's new in the physiopathology of acne? Br J Dermatol 2015;172(Suppl 1): 13–9.

45. Lai JJ, Chang P, Lai KP, et al. The role of androgen and androgen receptor in skin-related disorders. Arch Dermatol Res 2012;304(7):499–510.

46. Arora MK, Yadav A, Saini V. Role of hormones in acne vulgaris. Clin Biochem 2011;44(13):1035–40.

47. Simpson NB, Cunliffe WJ. Disorders of sebaceous glands. In: Burns T, Breatchnach S, Cox N, et al, editors. Rook's textbook of dermatology. 7th edition. Malden, MA: Blackwell Publishing Company; 2004. p. 43, 41-43.78.

48. Irwig MS. Testosterone therapy for transgender men. Lancet Diabetes Endocrinol 2016;5(4):301–11.

49. Wierckx K, Van de Peer F, Verhaeghe E, et al. Short- and long-term clinical skin effects of testosterone treatment in trans men. J Sex Med 2014;11(1): 222–9.

50. Park JA, Carter EE, Larson AR. Risk factors for acne development in the first 2 years after initiating masculinizing testosterone therapy among transgender men. J Am Acad Dermatol 2019;81(2): 617–8.

51. Burke BM, Cunliffe WJ. The assessment of acne vulgaris–the Leeds technique. Br J Dermatol 1984; 111(1):83–92.

52. Motosko CC, Zakhem GA, Pomeranz MK, et al. The impact of testosterone on the chests and abdomens of transgender men. J Am Acad Dermatol 2019; 81(2):634–6.

53. Motosko CC, Zakhem GA, Pomeranz MK, et al. Acne: a side-effect of masculinizing hormonal therapy in transgender patients. Br J Dermatol 2019; 180(1):26–30.

54. Ginsberg BA, Calderon M, Seminara NM, et al. A potential role for the dermatologist in the physical transformation of transgender people: a survey of attitudes and practices within the transgender community. J Am Acad Dermatol 2016;74(2):303–8.

55. Turrion-Merino L, Urech-Garcia-de-la-Vega M, Miguel-Gomez L, et al. Severe acne in female-to-male transgender patients. JAMA Dermatol 2015; 151(11):1260–1.

56. Campos-Munoz L, Lopez-De Lara D, Rodriguez-Rojo ML, et al. Transgender adolescents and acne: a cases series. Pediatr Dermatol 2018;35(3):e155–8.

57. Spring LK, Krakowski AC, Alam M, et al. Isotretinoin and timing of procedural interventions: a systematic review with consensus recommendations. JAMA Dermatol 2017;153(8):802–9.

58. US Food and Drug Administration Patient Information. 2016. Available at: https://www.ipledgeprogram.com/iPledgeUI/patientInfo.u. Accessed March 5, 2019.

59. Waldman RA, Waldman SD, Grant-Kels JM. The ethics of performing noninvasive, reversible gender-affirming procedures on transgender adolescents. J Am Acad Dermatol 2018;79(6):1166–8.

60. Yeung H, Chen SC, Katz KA, et al. Prescribing isotretinoin in the United States for transgender individuals: ethical considerations. J Am Acad Dermatol 2016;75(3):648–51.

61. Light A, Wang LF, Zeymo A, et al. Family planning and contraception use in transgender men. Contraception 2018;98(4):266–9.

62. Carswell JM, Roberts SA. Induction and maintenance of amenorrhea in transmasculine and nonbinary adolescents. Transgend Health 2017;2(1): 195–201.

63. Boos MD, Ginsberg BA, Peebles JK. Prescribing isotretinoin for transgender youth: a pledge for more inclusive care. Pediatr Dermatol 2019;36(1): 169–71.

64. Katz KA. Transgender patients, isotretinoin, and US Food and Drug Administration-mandated risk evaluation and mitigation strategies: a prescription for inclusion. JAMA Dermatol 2016;152(5):513–4.

65. George R, Clarke S, Thiboutot D. Hormonal therapy for acne. Semin Cutan Med Surg 2008;27(3): 188–96.

66. Thiboutot D. Acne: hormonal concepts and therapy. Clin Dermatol 2004;22(5):419–28.

67. Motosko CC, Pomeranz MK, Hazen A. Caught in a bind. JAMA Dermatol 2018;154(2):202.

68. Peitzmeier S, Gardner I, Weinand J, et al. Health impact of chest binding among transgender adults: a community-engaged, cross-sectional study. Cult Health Sex 2017;19(1):64–75.

69. Baumann L. Cosmetics and skin care in dermatology. In: Wolff K, Goldsmith L, Katz S, et al, editors. Fitzpatrick's dermatology in general medicine. 7 edition. New York McGraw Hill Medical; 2008. p. 2360.

Anogenital Dermatitis in Men Who Have Sex with Men

Patrick E. McCleskey, MD, FAAD

KEYWORDS

- LGBT • Male • Men who have sex with men • Dermatology • Irritant dermatitis
- Allergic contact dermatitis • Genital diseases, male • Anus diseases

KEY POINTS

- Patients with anogenital dermatitis should be asked about their sexual history because men who have sex with men have varying risk of certain infections.
- Focus history on personal products used by the patient and partner(s), including soaps, lotions, topical medications, personal lubricants, condoms, and any fragranced items.
- Irritant or allergic contact dermatitis often improves with avoidance of soaps, fragrances, preservatives, antibacterials, anesthetics, antifungals, antibiotics.
- Consider patch testing for standard tray plus antibiotics, antifungals, anesthetics, and topical steroids.
- Anal dermatitis may improve by switching to water washing, as well as removing irritants; limit anal douching to small amounts of plain water.

INTRODUCTION

Dermatitis of the penis, scrotum, or anus can be challenging to diagnose and treat, and in the case of men who have sex with men (MSM), or transgender women, dermatologists need to be aware of cultural and epidemiologic differences in this population. Although many transgender women have sex with men, not all do. This article mostly focuses on MSM, rather than transgender women. Many transgender women, however, never undergo gender affirmation surgery of the genitalia, and the epidemiology is similar for transgender women who have sex with men, and MSM. In general the same diagnoses and treatments are seen in the heterosexual population and sexual minorities, but there are a few differences to be aware of, including how we talk with patients.

It has been mentioned elsewhere that gathering sexual orientation and gender identity data as a standard practice can help LGBT (lesbian, gay, bisexual, transgender) patients feel more comfortable seeing a specialist because the practice demonstrates openness.[1,2] Addressing patients by their preferred names and pronouns is very important for caring for transgender patients. Although we must balance patient privacy with medical need, if a patient presents with a genital complaint, we must assess the genitalia present as well as surgical history, as appropriate. For instance, a transgender woman presented to our clinic last year for "vaginal itching" but review of her medical record showed the only gender affirmation surgery she had received was breast augmentation. The diagnosis was pruritus scroti, but she did not feel comfortable referring to her scrotum during the medical assistant's intake. This exemplifies the personal nature of the visit to the dermatologist when it comes to anogenital complaints. Setting the tone early and creating good rapport is essential. It is helpful to ask about privacy concerns and consider using chaperones whenever performing a genital examination.

Department of Dermatology, Kaiser Permanente, 3701 Broadway, Oakland, CA 94611, USA
E-mail address: Patrick.e.mccleskey@kp.org

Dermatol Clin 38 (2020) 227–232
https://doi.org/10.1016/j.det.2019.10.007
0733-8635/20/© 2019 Elsevier Inc. All rights reserved.

Choosing a more generic "pruritus" diagnosis, rather than "pruritus scroti," for example, is a show of respect for gender identity.

Genital dermatology complaints commonly include pruritus without rash. This article focuses on rashes of the penis and anus, as pruritus ani and pruritus scroti have been well reviewed elsewhere.[3,4]

There are some differences in the epidemiology of infectious dermatoses between MSM and men who have sex with women (MSW), so when evaluating a penile or perianal rash, it is appropriate to take a sexual history.[1,2] Ask if the patient has sex with men or women or both. Ask if they have a primary partner, and if they have sex with anyone other than their primary partner. If a man engages in sex with men and has more than one partner, identify risk behaviors, including whether they have receptive or insertive oral sex, and receptive or insertive anal sex. These behaviors affect their risk of developing chlamydia, gonorrhea, syphilis, herpes simplex virus (HSV), human papillomavirus (HPV), and human immunodeficiency virus (HIV). MSM with multiple partners should get routine screening for bacterial sexually transmitted infections (STIs) based on their behaviors.[1] This process of taking a sexual history provides an opportunity to discuss prevention measures, such as safer sex practices, vaccinations for hepatitis and HPV, and preexposure prophylaxis for HIV.

Incidence of the following infections is higher among MSM: HIV, genital herpes, HPV-induced anal cancer, hepatitis A and B, syphilis, chlamydia, gonorrhea, and possibly methicillin-resistant *Staphylococcus aureus*.[1] Many of these infections disproportionately affect the penis and anus, and may mimic dermatitis. Syphilis may rarely present with balanitis,[5,6] as can herpes simplex and *S aureus*. Balanitis also can be caused by group B streptococcus (GBS), and the incidence of GBS is increased in MSM.[7] Candida colonization is higher in MSM than MSW, but it also causes balanitis infrequently in MSM.[8] Other infectious causes of balanitis include group A streptococcus, *S aureus*, *Mycobacterium tuberculosis*, *Entamoeba histolytica*, HSV, and HPV.[5] Perianal infectious dermatitis is most commonly caused by group A streptococcus, but it also can be caused by GBS, group C streptococcus, group G streptococcus, *S aureus*, and *Enterococcus faecalis* in children.[9,10] GBS may be a more common cause in adults.[11] Scabies may cause itching of the anogenital region, but on the penis it classically presents as pruritic papules rather than balanitis. Dermoscopy allows for rapid, low-cost diagnosis of scabies.[12] For all these reasons, obtaining

serology for syphilis, viral culture or polymerase chain reaction–based swabs for HSV, and bacterial swabs for superficial bacteria or yeast, is important when evaluating a nonresponsive balanitis or anal dermatitis in MSM. In some cases, biopsy may be required to make a diagnosis of bacterial or viral infections.[13]

PENILE DERMATITIS

Dermatologists are very familiar with the common dermatoses of the penis,[14–16] which include seborrheic dermatitis, irritant contact dermatitis (ICD), allergic contact dermatitis (ACD), atopic dermatitis, psoriasis, lichen planus, lichen sclerosus, balanitis, fixed drug eruption, vitiligo, squamous cell carcinoma in situ and squamous cell carcinoma, Bowenoid papulosis, and infectious processes including warts, herpes, scabies, pediculosis, syphilis, molluscum contagiosum, candidiasis, and others. For many of these dermatoses, there is no clinical difference between MSM and MSW.

Once the possibility of an infectious cause of the dermatitis has been ruled out, other causes of dermatitis must be distinguished. In several case series of male genital dermatology clinics, the most common dermatosis was ICD.[13,17] Other common causes include lichen sclerosus, Zoon balanitis, nonspecific balanitis, atopic dermatitis, lichen planus, psoriasis, and seborrheic dermatitis.[15–18] In one series, 75% of cases were noninfectious balanitis, and the least common dermatoses were STIs (4%) and malignancies (9%).[18] Lichen sclerosus, infections, psoriasis, Zoon balanitis, balanoposthitis, seborrheic dermatitis, and all-cause penile dermatitis, were more common in uncircumcised than circumcised men.[15,17,18] Only lichen planus was more common in circumcised men.[18] Inflammatory dermatoses were more common in men with a history of atopy in 2 studies.[16,17] Most of these studies did not report separately on MSM compared with MSW. Only one of these studies mentions sexual behaviors and reported 5 of 43 men were homosexual.[16] Thus, there are few data available about possible differences in noninfectious dermatoses of the genitalia in MSM compared with MSW.

Lichen sclerosus, psoriasis, atopic dermatitis, lichen planus, and seborrheic dermatitis often have distinct presentations or other areas of the body that are involved. The correct diagnosis is usually found by a dermatologist through clinical examination or biopsy. Of note, patients are often recommended by nondermatologists to use topical antifungals before presenting to the dermatologist. As a result, selection bias may lead to lower rates of seborrheic dermatitis in clinical studies than in the general population.[16] When these more distinct dermatoses are set aside, noninfectious etiologies may be considered, including balanitis, Zoon balanitis, ICD, and ACD. The search for possible irritants and contact allergens becomes a critical component of making the correct diagnosis.

ICD of the penis may be caused by irritants such as soaps. One study found that frequent genital washing with soap or shower gel was associated with recurrent or unresponsive balanitis or nonspecific dermatitis of the penis. Avoidance of soaps and shower gels, as well as application of bland emollients and topical hydrocortisone, improved almost all the patients.[16] Studies on ACD specify ICD caused by iatrogenic substances such as 5-fluorouracil and podophyllin. Milder irritants included cleansers, soaps, bubble baths, douches, lubricants, personal wipes, urine, perspiration, feces, sanitary pads, clothing, and towels.[19–21] Many things coming in direct contact with the genitalia also may be irritating, such as urine (irritant ammonia dermatitis), topical medications, topical steroids, deodorants, hygiene sprays, metal, and clothing.[19] Irritant sources may be surfactants, preservatives, fragrances, ammonia, or adhesives. Men also may be overusing soaps after sex or masturbation, especially if they have a penile rash. Recommend using water only for cleansing or using soap alternatives or soaps with no preservatives, fragrances, or dyes, such as *Vanicream cleansing bar*, *Kiss My Face Pure Olive Oil Fragrance Free Soap*, and *Cleure Glycerin Face/Body SLS Free Bar Soap*.[20]

Patients often touch their hands to irritants then touch their anogenital region. Patients and their partners should provide an inventory of all the things that come into contact with their hands and genitalia, to help find possible irritants or allergens. One other possible irritant to be aware of is nitrates in the form of "poppers" that may be used to enhance anal sex. While "poppers dermatitis" generally involves the nares and face because they are inhaled, it can rarely irritate the genitalia through inadvertent contact or partner contact.[22]

LUBRICANTS AND CONDOMS

As with MSW, MSM may have ICD from personal lubricants, or friction during sex or masturbation. Dermatologists should therefore inquire about the use and brand of lubricants and condoms. For instance, some men use desensitizing lubricants for anal sex to avoid premature ejaculation. These may contain benzocaine or lidocaine,

possible causes of ACD of the penis or anus of the insertive or receptive partner. Water-based lubricants also may contain well-known allergens, such as parabens, chlorhexidine, propylene glycol, quaternium 15, and fragrances. For very sensitive patients, silicone-based lubricants generally have fewer preservatives. Dimethicone, the most common primary ingredient in silicone-based lubricants, is not generally implicated as a cause of anogenital dermatitis. Patients should look for silicone-based lubricants with the fewest number of ingredients, such as Uberlube or Mr. S Bodyglide Premium Silicone Lube. For those who cannot tolerate silicone-based lubricants, alternative water-based lubricants that are less likely to irritate include Sliquid Naturals H2O Lubricant and Wet Naturals Gel Lubricant.[20]

Condoms also can cause ICD or ACD on the penis. Causes of ACD from condoms include latex, rubber sensitizers (thiurams, mercaptobenzthiazole), topical anesthetics (benzocaine, lidocaine), fragrances, colors, and spermicides (nonoxynol-9).[19,23–25] True latex allergy, a type I hypersensitivity reaction, is uncommon. If patients suspect true latex allergy, skin prick testing or immunoglobulin (Ig)E-specific antibody testing (enzyme-linked immunosorbent assay or radioallergosorbent testing) can be performed.[23] A brief wear test, also called the glove provocation test, with wear of a single finger of a latex glove, then the whole glove, under supervision of an allergist in case of an anaphylactic reaction, also can be used to test for latex allergy. If skin prick, IgE testing, wear test, and patch testing are all negative, the likely cause is ICD from personal lubricants or friction from lack of lubricant use. Patients with ICD of the penis should use small amounts of lubricant before donning condoms to reduce friction. For patients with ACD to rubber, polyurethane or polyisoprene condoms may be a good alternative.[20]

ANOGENITAL ALLERGIC CONTACT DERMATITIS

When it comes to patch-test–proven ACD, men with anogenital dermatitis reportedly have more relevant patch test reactions than women.[21] Fragrances are the most common culprits in anogenital ACD, with relevant positive patch testing in as many as 20% of anogenital ACD cases.[20,21] Fragrance may be found in lubricants, condoms, soaps, douches, laundry detergent, perfumes and colognes, cosmetics, lotions, sanitary or incontinence pads, toilet paper, wipes, and many other products. Connubial contact dermatitis is when ACD arises from contact with the skin of a partner. Fragrances on a partner's face, hands, or genitalia also may be the cause of anogenital dermatitis.[19] Preservatives also cause anogenital ACD, including methylchloroisothiazolinone (MCI), methylisothiazolinone (MI), formaldehyde releasers, benzalkonium chloride, methyldibromo glutaronitrile, thimerosal, and multiple parabens. Formaldehyde releasers and dyes can contribute to ACD from clothing. Vehicles including isopropyl myristate, ethylenediamine, propylene glycol, octyldodecanol, and lanolin also can cause ACD.

Topical preparations frequently applied to the genital area may undergo sensitization.[19–21,26] These include local anesthetics (benzocaine, dibucaine, lidocaine, tetracaine), topical corticosteroids (triamcinolone, tixocortol, hydrocortisone, budesonide), topical antibiotics (neomycin, bacitracin), topical antifungals (eg, terconazole, miconazole, econazole, clotrimazole), and nonsteroidal anti-inflammatories (bufexamac was used in the past for anal eczema and hemorrhoids).

Contact dermatitis experts suggest adding topical anesthetics, topical antibiotics, and topical antifungals to standard patch test trays in cases of anogenital dermatitis.[20,21,26] When it is not possible to test for additional allergens, an open application test with any leave-on product is a good alternative.

ANAL DERMATITIS

Perianal dermatitis can be infectious, but more often it is irritant. Dermatologists frequently see patients with anal itching without rash, and similar educational principles apply with regard to irritant avoidance.[3,4,27] As with balanitis, washing with soaps can be very irritating. Furthermore, preservatives are a frequent source of irritant or allergic contact dermatitis. Moist towelettes or wipes often contain propylene glycol, MCI, or MI, all of which can cause ACD.[28] Patients should avoid moist wipes in favor of damp cotton wash clothes or dampened paper towels without inked patterns. For instance, *Viva*, is reportedly stronger than others and does not have added fragrances. For parents or patients who cannot avoid using wipes, some dermatologists recommend *Water Wipes Baby Wipes*, which contain only water and 0.002% benzalkonium chloride via a minute amount of grapefruit seed extract. These wipes may be less likely to cause irritation except in the most exquisitely sensitive patients to benzalkonium chloride.[29] Switching from toilet paper to using a bidet to wash after defecation improves symptoms in up to 60% of patients with anal dermatitis.[27] Use of bidets may be slowly gaining acceptance in the United States,[30] and home bidet kits are relatively inexpensive, making this an increasingly available option to patients with anal dermatitis.

In addition to asking MSM patients with anal dermatitis about toilet hygiene practices, one must also ask about sexual practices, as mentioned previously. Types of lubricants used, condoms used, toys inserted into the anus, and gloves or specialized lubricants used in anal fisting, could all potentially contribute to anal dermatitis if applicable to that patient. Men who engage in receptive anal sex should be asked about anal cleansing practices, also known as enemas or douching. Methylparabens and sodium benzoate in some douches may cause ACD.[31] Some MSM mix soap with water when douching, and this can be a possible irritant as well that may go unrecognized if the dermatologist does not inquire about it. Most men, however, prefer warm water alone to prepare for receptive anal intercourse, and a small amount of plain water is probably the safest method of anal douching.[32] Overuse of sodium phosphate enemas used for anal douching also can cause kidney damage.[33]

Most patients with anogenital dermatitis will improve once irritants are removed, and possible allergic contact dermatitis is addressed.[16,27] When this is insufficient, low-potency topical corticosteroids can control symptoms when used for short periods. If symptoms worsen with topical steroids, ACD to steroids should be considered, and calcineurin inhibitors may be appropriate alternatives. For anogenital dermatitis that is not responsive to measures of avoiding irritants and use of topical steroids, biopsy must be considered to rule out neoplasia or help aid in diagnosis. Small biopsies (2-mm snip biopsies or 3-mm punch biopsies) are generally well tolerated.

For MSM patients with anogenital dermatitis, consideration of possible infections and contribution of hygiene and sexual practices is essential for complete care and counseling. Although many anogenital dermatoses are the same regardless of sexual orientation or behavior, open engagement with our patients, including asking about sexual practices as appropriate, provides better overall dermatologic care and improved quality of life.

SUMMARY

Men who have sex with men who present with anogenital rashes should be evaluated with a thorough history including sexual practices, use of topical products, and partners' products. Once infectious etiologies have been considered and tested for as appropriate, counseling on avoidance of irritants often helps lead to symptom improvement (**Box 1**). Low potency

---

Box 1
Tips for anogenital dermatitis in men who have sex with men

- Take a sexual history, including whether the patient has receptive or insertive oral sex and anal sex. Ask about use of condoms, lubricants, poppers, or other sexual enhancements. Ask about products their partner(s) may be using as well.
- When reviewing possible infectious etiologies and sexually transmitted infections (STIs), consider whether additional testing is necessary (syphilis serologies, urethral throat or rectal tests for chlamydia and gonorrhea, human immunodeficiency virus testing), based on the patient's sexual behaviors since their last STI testing.
- Skin cultures for bacterial, yeast, and viral causes may be indicated.
- Stop using all home remedies, topical medications, and hygiene wipes.
- Avoid cleaning with soap in the affected area, or use only use low-irritant soaps without fragrances, dyes, or preservatives,
- Use fragrance-free laundry detergent, moisturizers, and so forth. Avoid colognes.
  - Cleansers recommended by the American Contact Dermatitis Society (ACDS): Kiss My Face Pure Olive Oil Soap Fragrance Free, Cleure Glycerin Face/Body SLS Free Bar Soap
  - Detergents recommend by ACDS: Greenshield Organic Free and Clear detergent, The Honest Company detergent
- Use only plain Vaseline for moisturizer after showers.
- Avoid anal douching with anything other than water.
- Use water washing rather than toilet paper or wipes, or use a damp paper towel or gentle washcloth after defecating.
- Consider using silicone-based lubricants with the fewest number of ingredients, no fragrance, parabens, or glycerin.
  - Water-based lubricants recommended by ACDS: Sliquid Naturals H2O Lubricant, Wet Naturals Gel Lubricant
  - Silicone-based lubricants with few ingredients: Uberlube, Mr S Bodyglide Premium Silicone Lube
- Use low-dose steroid ointments to control symptoms if needed.
- If not responsive to avoidance and topical steroids or calcineurin inhibitors, consider biopsy.

Adapted from Yale K, Asowika O, Rengifo-Pardo M, Ehrlich A. Genital allergic contact dermatitis. Dermatitis. 2018;29(3):112-119.

---

steroid ointments are often needed for intermittent use. Less commonly, patch testing may reveal a source, and rarely, biopsy may be needed to rule out infectious or neoplastic causes.

DISCLOSURE

I have no relationship with a commercial company that has a direct financial interest in subject matter or materials discussed in article or with a company making a competing product.

REFERENCES

1. Yeung H, Luk KM, Chen SC, et al. Dermatologic care of lesbian, gay, bisexual, and transgender persons. J Am Acad Dermatol 2018;80(3): 591–602.

2. Charny JW, Kovarik CL. LGBT access to health care: a dermatologist's role in building a therapeutic relationship. Cutis 2017;99:228–9.

3. Weichert GE. An approach to the treatment of anogenital pruritus. Dermatol Ther 2004;17(1):129–33.

4. Zuccati G, Lotti T, Mastrolorenzo A, et al. Pruritus ani. Dermatol Ther 2005;18(4):355–62.

5. Edwards S. Balanitis and balanoposthitis: a review. Genitourin Med 1996;72:155–9.

6. Zubair R, Chen W, Khera P. A protean master mimic: secondary syphilis presenting as psoriasiform balanitis. J Am Acad Dermatol 2016;74(5):AB149.

7. Bhargava RK, Thin RNT. Subpreputial carriage of aerobic micro-organisms and balanitis. Br J Vener Dis 1983;59:131–3.

8. David LM, Walzman M, Rajamanoharan S. Genital colonisation and infection with candida in heterosexual and homosexual males. Genitourin Med 1997; 73:394–6.

9. Patrizi A, Costa AM, Fiorillo L, et al. Perianal strepto-coccal dermatitis associated with guttate psoriasis and/or balanoposthitis: a study of five cases. Pediatr Dermatol 1994;11:168–71.

10. Serban ED. Perianal infectious dermatitis: an under-diagnosed, unremitting and stubborn condition. World J Clin Pediatr 2018;7(4):89–104.

11. Kahlke V, Jongen J, Peleikis HG, et al. Perianal streptococcal dermatitis in adults: its association with pruritic anorectal diseases is mainly caused by group B Streptococci. Colorectal Dis 2013; 15(5):602–7.

12. Prins C, Stuck L, French L, et al. Dermoscopy for the in vivo detection of Sarcoptes scabiei. Dermatology 2004;208:241–3.

13. Birley HDL, Walker MM, Luzzi GA, et al. Clinical fea-tures and management of recurrent balanitis; asso-ciation with atopy and genital washing. Genitourin Med 1993;69(5):400–3.

14. Buechner SA. Common skin disorders of the penis. BJU Int 2002;90(5):498–506.

15. Mallon E, Hawkins D, Dinneen M, et al. Circumcision and genital dermatoses. Arch Dermatol 2000;136: 350–4.

16. Van Dijk F, Thio HB, Neumann HAM. Non-oncolog-ical and non-infectious disease of the penis. Eur As-soc Urol 2006;4:13–9.

17. Elakis JA, Hall AP. Skin disease of penis and male genitalia is linked to atopy and circumcision: case-load in a male genital dermatology clinic. Australas J Dermatol 2017;58(3):e68–72.

18. Shaw M. Clinical outcomes in a specialist male gen-ital skin clinic: prospective follow-up of 600 patients. Clin Exp Dermatol 2017;42(7):723–7.

19. Marfatia YS, Patel D, Menon DS, et al. Genital con-tact allergy: a diagnosis missed. Indian J Sex Trams Dis AIDS 2016;37(1):1–6.

20. Yale K, Asowika O, Rengifo-Pardo M, et al. Genital allergic contact dermatitis. Dermatitis 2018;29(3): 112–9.

21. Warshaw EM, Furda LM, Maiback HI, et al. Anogen-ital dermatitis in patients referred for patch testing. Arch Dermatol 2008;144(6):749–55.

22. Latini A, Lora V, Zaccarelli M, et al. Unusual presen-tation of poppers dermatitis. JAMA Dermatol 2017; 153(2):233–4.

23. Burkhart C, Schloemer J, Zirwas M. Differentiation between latex allergy and irritant contact dermatitis. Cutis 2015;96:369–71, 401.

24. Nettis E. Contact allergy to benzocaine in a condom. Contact Dermatitis 2008;59:173–4.

25. Fisher AA. Allergic contact dermatitis to nonoxynol-9 in a condom. Cutis 1994;53:110–1.

26. Bauer A, Oehme S, Geier J. Contact sensitization in the anal and genital area. Curr Probl Dermatol 2011; 40:133–41.

27. Havlickova B, Weyandt GH. Therapeutic manage-ment of anal eczema: an evidence-based review. Int J Clin Pract 2014;68(11):1388–99.

28. Gardner KH, David MDP, Richardson DM, et al. The hazards of moist toilet paper: allergy to the preser-vative methylchloroisothiazolinone/methylisothiazoli-none. Arch Dermatol 2010;146(8):886–90.

29. Water wipes baby wipes. Available at: https://www.waterwipes.com/us/en/health-care. Accessed April 2, 2019.

30. The bidet's revival, The Atlantic. Available at: https://www.theatlantic.com/technology/archive/2018/03/the-bidets-revival/555770/. Accessed April 2, 2019.

31. Raulin-Gaignard H, Berlegni N, Gatin A, et al. Se-vere allergic reaction due to a rectal enema. Arch Pediatr 2013;20(12):1329–32 [in French].

32. Carballo-Dieguez A, Lentz C, Giguere R. Rectal douching associated with receptive anal inter-course: a literature review. AIDS Behav 2018;22(4): 1288–94.

33. FDA Drug Safety Communication. Available at: https://www.fda.gov/downloads/drugs/drugsafety/ucm381084.pdf. Accessed Apr 2, 2019.

Preexposure Prophylaxis for Human Immunodeficiency Virus Infection for Men Who Have Sex with Men and Transgender Persons:
What Dermatologists Need to Know

Kenneth A. Katz, MD, MSc, MSCE[a],*, Andrew J. Park, MD[b],
Julia L. Marcus, PhD, MPH[c]

KEYWORDS

- HIV • Men who have sex with men • Transgender • PrEP • Prevention

KEY POINTS

- The ongoing HIV epidemic in the United States disproportionately affects men who have sex with men (MSM) and transgender persons, particularly members of racial/ethnic minority groups.
- Preexposure prophylaxis for HIV, called PrEP, is an HIV prevention approach in which persons who are HIV-uninfected take antiretroviral medications during periods with potential HIV exposures to reduce risk of HIV infection.
- PrEP has been shown to be very effective in preventing HIV infection when taken orally daily or, for some persons, intermittently, with few adverse effects.
- Patient and provider barriers to PrEP uptake exist for MSM and transgender persons.
- Dermatologists should know how, when, and why PrEP should be considered for MSM and transgender persons at high risk of HIV infection.

INTRODUCTION

In the early 1980s, outbreaks of Kaposi sarcoma (KS) and *Pneumocystis carinii* pneumonia among gay men heralded the beginning of the HIV/AIDS epidemic.[1–3] In subsequent years, dermatologists played a crucial role in describing and treating KS and other mucocutaneous opportunistic infections in persons living with, and too often dying from, HIV infection.[4–7]

Nearly 40 years later, HIV remains an important public health issue in the United States and throughout the world.[8,9] In the United States, the epidemic has and continues to disproportionately affect gay men and other men who have sex with men (hereafter collectively called MSM) and transgender women. In the United States, MSM accounted for 67% of 38,281 new HIV infections in 2017; 55% of persons living with HIV infection in 2016; 42% of deaths of persons with diagnosed

a Department of Dermatology, Kaiser Permanente, 1600 Owens Street, 9th Floor, San Francisco, CA 94158, USA; b Department of Medicine, Kaiser Permanente Oakland Medical Center, 3600 Broadway, Oakland, CA 94611, USA; c Department of Population Medicine, Harvard Medical School, Harvard Pilgrim Health Care Institute, Boston, MA 02215, USA
* Corresponding author.
E-mail address: Kenneth.Katz@gmail.com

Dermatol Clin 38 (2020) 233–238
https://doi.org/10.1016/j.det.2019.10.008

HIV infection in 2016; and 47% of deaths of persons with diagnosed HIV infection ever classified as having AIDS since the beginning of the epidemic.[10] (Including MSM who inject drugs brings those figures to 70%, 60%, 51%, and 55%, respectively.) Less well tracked is HIV prevalence among transgender women and men in the United States, estimated to be 14.1% and 3.2%, respectively.[11] Substantial disparities exist by race, ethnicity, gender, and geography in HIV incidence, prevalence, and outcomes in the United States, including among MSM and transgender persons.[10]

For much of the epidemic, prevention strategies have focused on reducing risk of HIV infection by encouraging behavioral changes among at-risk populations, such as having sex with condoms, limiting numbers of sexual partners, and adopting safer injection-drug-use practices. With the emergence of effective antiretroviral treatment, treatment of individuals living with HIV to prevent transmission, and postexposure prophylaxis for persons exposed to HIV to prevent acquisition, have also been adopted as approaches to combat the epidemic.[12]

In the past decade, another approach has emerged: preexposure prophylaxis for HIV, commonly called PrEP (preexposure prophylaxis), in which persons uninfected with HIV take anti-HIV medications during periods with potential HIV exposures to reduce HIV infection risk.

Dermatologists should learn about PrEP for 2 reasons. First, dermatologists should understand why persons uninfected with HIV might be taking anti-HIV medications. Second, dermatologists should know when and how to refer patients for consideration of PrEP. To those ends, this article reviews PrEP's effectiveness; adverse effects of PrEP; indications for taking PrEP; and PrEP uptake. The article's scope is limited to PrEP among MSM and transgender persons in the United States. Additionally, the article was written prior to FDA approval, on October 3, 2019, of emtricitabine and tenofovir alafenamide (Descovy) for PrEP to reduce the risk of HIV-1 infection from sexual acquisition, excluding individuals at risk from receptive vaginal sex, and to the U.S. Preventive Services Task Force's issuance, in July 2019, of its final recommendation on PrEP, which endorsed the draft recommendations discussed below.

EFFECTIVENESS OF PREEXPOSURE PROPHYLAXIS

The most commonly used PrEP regimen in the United States involves taking a single daily pill containing 2 antiretroviral medicines—emtricitabine 200 mg and tenofovir disoproxil fumarate 300 mg. The brand name of the combination pill, commonly used by persons taking it, is Truvada.

A randomized clinical trial (RCT) studied the effectiveness of emtricitabine-tenofovir, taken daily, compared with placebo among MSM and transgender women.[13] Both groups received safer sex messaging, including regarding consistent condom use. Results of the trial, published in the New England Journal of Medicine in 2010, showed a 44% decrease in HIV infection among participants taking emtricitabine-tenofovir compared with participants taking placebo. Among participants taking emtricitabine-tenofovir who were compliant (defined as having detectable drug levels), the decrease was even more pronounced: 92%. A subgroup analysis of transgender women in the trial did not show a statistically significant decrease in HIV infection, possibly from lower compliance rates.[14,15]

The pill's manufacturer subsequently applied to the US Food and Drug Administration (FDA) for approval for prevention of HIV infection. Approval was granted in 2012 "in combination with safer sex practices for preexposure prophylaxis to reduce risk of sexually acquired HIV-1 in at-risk adults." Daily emtricitabine-tenofovir remains the only FDA-approved PrEP regimen.[16,17] In May 2018, FDA approved use of daily emtricitabine-tenofovir in adolescents weighing $\geq$35 kg.[16]

In real-world settings, daily emtricitabine-tenofovir has been extremely effective in preventing HIV infection. Among 4991 PrEP users in Northern California, for example, not a single infection occurred during 5104 person-years of PrEP use.[18] Only 6 HIV infections in persons taking daily emtricitabine-tenofovir for PrEP have been reported; all resulted from HIV strains resistant to tenofovir or emtricitabine.[19]

An alternative PrEP regimen has more recently been endorsed by an expert panel[20] and others[21,22] for MSM at substantial risk of HIV infection from sexual exposure but who are unable or would prefer not to take daily emtricitabine-tenofovir. The alternative regimen—commonly called "2-1-1"—involves taking 2 emtricitabine-tenofovir tablets 2 hours before anticipated sexual exposure, followed by single tablets 24 and 48 hours postexposure. In an RCT conducted among MSM, 2-1-1 reduced HIV infection by 86% compared with placebo.[23] 2-1-1 has not been approved by FDA or endorsed by the Centers for Disease Control and Prevention (CDC) and is not yet recommended for other groups at high risk of HIV infection, including transgender persons, injection drug users, and persons infected with the hepatitis B virus.[20]

Other PrEP regimens, including oral, intramuscular, and topical formulations, are in development.[24]

ADVERSE EFFECTS OF PREEXPOSURE PROPHYLAXIS

Concerns about PrEP have focused on adverse effects of medication and potential changes in sexual behaviors among PrEP users that might increase risk of infection by other sexually transmitted infections (STIs).

Regarding adverse effects from medications, a systematic review of RCTs studying daily emtricitabine-tenofovir for PrEP found no significant differences in adverse events between active and placebo groups.[25] Gastrointestinal adverse effects, including nausea and diarrhea, required PrEP interruptions in some persons, most of whom subsequently reinitiated PrEP without recurrence of those effects.[25] Subclinical changes in renal and hepatic function and bone mineral density have occurred in some RCTs.[26] In real-world settings, adverse events have rarely led to PrEP discontinuation.[27] CDC guidelines include recommendations for pre-PrEP testing and counseling and for adverse event monitoring.[17]

Concerns regarding changes in sexual behavior stem from a concept called "risk compensation," in which persons who feel protected from a harm might engage in behaviors that put them at risk of other harms. Some data suggest that, among MSM using PrEP, STI rates are high,[28] although valid comparison groups are lacking.[29] Concerns about risk compensation, however, should not preclude prescribing of PrEP, because the benefits of preventing HIV infection outweigh potential harms.[30]

PREEXPOSURE PROPHYLAXIS INDICATIONS

CDC first issued clinical guidelines for PrEP in 2014, with an update issued in 2017.[17] PrEP indications for men who have sex only with men, according to the 2017 guidelines, are as follows:

- Adult man
- Without acute or established HIV infection
- Any male sex partners in past 6 months
- Not in a monogamous partnership with a recently tested, HIV-negative man

AND at least one of the following:

- Any anal sex without condoms (receptive or insertive) in past 6 months

- A bacterial STI (syphilis, gonorrhea, or chlamydia) diagnosed or reported in past 6 months[17]

CDC guidelines also include separate PrEP indications for MSM who also have sex with women and/or inject drugs.[17] A 2015 CDC study estimated that 24.7% of sexually active MSM in the United States—or 813,970 MSM—met indications for PrEP.[31,32]

CDC guidelines do not include specific PrEP indications for transgender persons but recommend consideration of PrEP in transgender persons who are at risk of sexual acquisition of HIV.[17]

Notably for dermatologists, a diagnosis of syphilis—which has many mucocutaneous manifestations and disproportionately affects MSM[33]—is one indication for PrEP. Syphilis among HIV-uninfected MSM and transgender women correlates with substantial risk of subsequent HIV infection.[34]

In November 2018, the US Preventive Services Task Force—a panel that makes clinical preventive services recommendations—released its first draft recommendation regarding daily emtricitabine-tenofovir for PrEP.[35] The draft recommended PrEP for HIV-uninfected persons at high risk of HIV infection, including MSM with one of the following characteristics:

- A serodiscordant sex partner (ie, a sex partner living with HIV)
- A recent STI with syphilis, gonorrhea, or chlamydia
- Inconsistent use of condoms during receptive or insertive anal sex

The draft also recommended PrEP for transgender persons at high risk of HIV infection.[35]

The draft recommendation carries an A grade, meaning the panel believes with high certainty that net benefit is substantial.[36] An A grade on a final recommendation would also mean, under the Affordable Care Act, that health insurers must cover PrEP for persons covered by the recommendation without cost-sharing (ie, copays or deductibles).[37]

PREEXPOSURE PROPHYLAXIS UPTAKE

Daily PrEP use is increasing in the United States, with 78,360 users aged ≥16 years taking daily PrEP for >30 days in 2016 compared with 13,748 in 2014.[38] Of users in 2016, 95% were men; MSM status was not reported. Given the estimate that greater than 800,000 MSM meet PrEP criteria,[31] substantial barriers to PrEP uptake clearly remain.

Stark racial, ethnic, gender, and geographic disparities in PrEP uptake also exist.[33] For example, although black men and women comprised approximately 40% of persons meeting PrEP indications in 1 study, white men and women were 6 times more likely to be prescribed PrEP than black men and women.[33] Notably, racial and ethnic disparities in PrEP uptake exist even in insured populations with access to care.[39]

Barriers to PrEP uptake exist for both patients and providers. Among MSM, barriers include lack of PrEP awareness, cost and insurance concerns, perceived low risk of HIV infection, concerns about medication side effects, and culturally insensitive care, and—more so among black than white MSM—medical mistrust and anti-gay and anti-HIV stigma.[40,41] Barriers among transgender women include concerns about side effects, difficulty taking pills, stigma, exclusion of transgender women in PrEP-related advertising, and lack of research on transgender women and PrEP.[42] Barriers among transgender men include possible side effects, cost issues, identifying trans-competent providers, importance of contraception, and condom use.[43]

Regarding cost, the list price of daily emtricitabine-tenofovir is nearly $2000 per month.[44] Many insurance plans help cover costs, although deductibles and copays can hinder access to PrEP.[27,45] The manufacturer of emtricitabine-tenofovir has programs that can help defray costs for insured, uninsured, or underinsured persons.[46] Two factors might reduce costs in the future. First, a generic version of the medicine is expected to be available in September 2020. Second, the U.S. government filed a lawsuit in November 2019 alleging that the medicine's manufacturer infringed PrEP-related patents belonging to the government (https://www.hhs.gov/about/news/2019/11/06/us-files-patent-infringement-lawsuit-against-gilead-pre-exposure-prophylaxis-hiv.html).

The knowledge, attitudes, and practices of dermatologists regarding PrEP have not been studied. Among other physicians, barriers to PrEP prescribing include time constraints; lack of familiarity with and knowledge about PrEP; uncertainty about insurance coverage; ambiguity about who should prescribe PrEP; lack of comfort with discussing sexual activities, testing for acute HIV, or conveying a new HIV diagnosis; and concerns about risk compensation.[47–49] Lack of risk-assessment tools to identify patients at risk of HIV infection is another obstacle.[50]

Dermatologists can help overcome some of those barriers to help mitigate some disparities in PrEP uptake by becoming familiar with PrEP and those patients who might benefit from it. Although dermatologists themselves might not be prescribing PrEP, they can and should refer to providers who are prepared to prescribe it. An Internet-based CDC database that identifies location-specific providers who offer PrEP is available to dermatologists and other providers as well as members of the public.[51]

SUMMARY

PrEP is a critically important HIV prevention approach for HIV-uninfected MSM and transgender persons. By understanding why, when, and how PrEP can be used for HIV prevention, dermatologists can help mitigate the disproportionate impact of the ongoing HIV epidemic on MSM and transgender persons.

DISCLOSURE

K.A. Katz and A.J. Park have nothing to disclose. J.L. Marcus received a research grant support from Merck and has consulted on a research grant to Kaiser Permanente Northern California from Gilead Sciences.

REFERENCES

1. Centers for Disease Control. Pneumocystis pneumonia—Los Angeles. MMWR Morb Mortal Wkly Rep 1981;30:250–2.
2. Centers for Disease Control. Kaposi's sarcoma and *Pneumocystis* pneumonia among homosexual men—New York City and California. MMWR Morb Mortal Wkly Rep 1981;30:305–8.
3. Centers for Disease Control. A cluster of Kaposi's sarcoma and *Pneumocystis carinii* pneumonia among homosexual male residents of Los Angeles and Orange Counties, California. MMWR Morb Mortal Wkly Rep 1982;31:305–7. Available at: https://www.cdc.gov/mmwr/preview/mmwrhtml/00001114.htm. Accessed March 6, 2019.
4. Friedman-Kien AE. Disseminated Kaposi's sarcoma syndrome in young homosexual men. J Am Acad Dermatol 1981;5:468–71.
5. Conant MA. AIDS and Kaposi's sarcoma. Curr Probl Dermatol 1985;13:92–108.
6. Kaplan MH, Sadic N, McNutt NS, et al. Dermatologic findings and manifestations of acquired immunodeficiency syndrome (AIDS). J Am Acad Dermatol 1987;16:485–506.
7. Tschachler E. The dermatologists and the HIV/AIDS pandemic. Clin Dermatol 2014;32(2):286–9.
8. The White House. National HIV/AIDS Strategy for the United States: updated to 2020. 2015. Available at: https://files.hiv.gov/s3fs-public/nhas-update.pdf. Accessed March 6, 2019.

9. World Health Organization. Global health sector strategy on HIV, 2016-2021. 2016. Available at: https://apps.who.int/iris/bitstream/handle/10665/246 178/WHO-HIV-2016.05-eng.pdf;jsessionid=66DB90 518FBD22B96A7CF61550321533?sequence=1. Accessed March 6, 2019.

10. Centers for Disease Control and Prevention. HIV surveillance report, 2017; vol. 29. 2018. Available at: https://www.cdc.gov/hiv/pdf/library/reports/surveillance/cdc-hiv-surveillance-report-2017-vol-29.pdf. Accessed March 28, 2019.

11. Becasen JS, Denard CL, Mullins MM, et al. Estimating the prevalence of HIV and sexual behaviors among the US transgender population: a systematic review and meta-analysis, 2006–2017. Am J Public Health 2018;e1–8. https://doi.org/10.2105/AJPH. 2018.304727.

12. CDC. Prevention. Available at: https://www.cdc.gov/hiv/basics/prevention.html. Accessed April 3, 2019.

13. Grant RM, Lama JR, Anderson PL, et al. Preexposure chemoprophylaxis for HIV prevention in men who have sex with men. N Engl J Med 2010;363: 2587–99.

14. Deutsch MB, Glidden DV, Sevelius J, et al. HIV preexposure prophylaxis in transgender women: a subgroup analysis of the iPREx trial. Lancet HIV 2015;2: e512–9.

15. Marshall BDL, Mimiaga MJ. Uptake and effectives of PrEP for transgender women. Lancet HIV 2015;2: e502–3.

16. Truvada label. Available at: https://dailymed.nlm.nih. gov/dailymed/drugInfo.cfm?setid=54e82b13-a037-49ed-b4b3-030b37c0ecdd. Accessed March 28, 2019.

17. Centers for Disease Control and Prevention. US Public Health Service: preexposure prophylaxis for the prevention of HIV infection in the United States— 2017 Update: a clinical practice guideline. 2018. Available at: https://www.cdc.gov/hiv/pdf/risk/prep/cdc-hiv-prep-guidelines-2017.pdf. Accessed March 28, 2019.

18. Marcus JL, Hurley LB, Nguyen DP, et al. Redefining human immunodeficiency virus (HIV) preexposure prophylaxis failures. Clin Infect Dis 2017;65: 1768–9.

19. Cohen SE, Sachdev D, Lee S, et al. Acquisition of TDF-susceptible HIV despite high level adherence to daily TDF/FTC PrEP as measured by dried blood spot (DBS) and segmental hair analysis: a case report. Poster 1298. IDWeek 2018. Available at: https://idsa.confex.com/idsa/2018/webprogram/Paper69862.html. Accessed April 2, 2019.

20. Saag MS, Benson CA, Gandhi RT. Antiretroviral drugs for treatment and prevention of HIV infection in adults: 2018 recommendations of the international antiviral society-USA panel. JAMA 2018; 320:379–96.

21. San Francisco Department of Public Health. Important HIV prevention and treatment updates for San Francisco providers. 2019. Available at: http://www.sfcityclinic.org/providers/HIVUpdate_02122019_v2.pdf. Accessed April 2, 2019.

22. Bajko MS. SF health officials embrace non-daily PrEP dosing regimen. The Bay Area Reporter. 2019. Available at: https://www.ebar.com/news/news/272877/sf_health_officials_embrace_non-daily_prep_dosing_regimen_. Accessed April 2, 2019.

23. Molina JM, Capitant C, Spire B, et al. On-demand preexposure prophylaxis in men at high risk for HIV-1 infection. N Engl J Med 2015;373:2237–46.

24. Hendrix CW. HIV antiretroviral pre-exposure prophylaxis: development challenges and pipeline promise. Clin Pharmacol Ther 2018;104:1082–97.

25. Fonner VA, Dalglish SL, Kennedy CE, et al. Effectiveness and safety of oral HIV preexposure prophylaxis for all populations. AIDS 2016;30:1973–83.

26. Mulligan K, Glidden DV, Anderson PL, et al. Effects of emtricitabine/tenofovir on bone mineral density in HIV-negative persons in a randomized, double-blind, placebo-controlled trial. Clin Infect Dis 2015; 61:572–80.

27. Marcus JL, Hurley LB, Hare CB, et al. Preexposure prophylaxis for HIV prevention in a large integrated health care system: adherence, renal safety, and discontinuation. J Acquir Immune Defic Syndr 2016;73:540–6.

28. Volk JE, Marcus JL, Phengrasamy T, et al. No new HIV infections with increasing use of HIV preexposure prophylaxis in a clinical practice setting. Clin Infect Dis 2015;61:1601–3.

29. Marcus JL, Volk JE, Snowden JM. Concerns about a study on sexually transmitted infections after initiation of HIV preexposure prophylaxis. AIDS 2018; 32:955–6.

30. Marcus JL, Katz KA, Krakower DS, et al. Risk compensation and clinical decision making—the case of HIV preexposure prophylaxis. N Engl J Med 2019;380:510–2.

31. Smith DK, Van Handel M, Wolitski RJ, et al. Vital signs: estimated percentages and numbers of adults with indications for preexposure prophylaxis to prevent HIV acquisition—United States, 2015. MMWR Morb Mortal Wkly Rep 2015;64:1291–5.

32. Smith DK, Van Handel M, Grey J, et al. Estimates of adults with indications for HIV pre-exposure prophylaxis by jurisdiction, transmission risk group, and race/ethnicity, United States, 2015. Ann Epidemiol 2018;28:850–7.e9.

33. Centers for Disease Control and Prevention. Sexually transmitted disease surveillance 2017. Atlanta (GA): U.S. Department of Health and Human Services; 2018. Available at: https://www.cdc.gov/std/stats17/2017-STD-Surveillance-Report_CDC-clearance-9.10. 18.pdf. Accessed April 2, 2019.

34. Solomon MM, Mayer KH, Glidden DV, et al. Syphilis predicts HIV incidence among men and transgender women who have sex with men in a preexposure prophylaxis trial. Clin Infect Dis 2014;59: 1020–6.

35. U.S. Preventive Services. Task Force. Draft recommendation statement. Prevention of human immunodeficiency virus (HIV) infection: pre-exposure prophylaxis. Available at: https://www.uspreventiveservicestaskforce.org/Page/Document/draft-recommendation-statement/prevention-of-human-immunodeficiency-virus-hiv-infection-pre-exposure-prophylaxis. Accessed April 2, 2019.

36. U.S. Preventive Services. Task force. Grade definitions. Available at: https://www.uspreventiveservicestaskforce.org/Page/Name/grade-definitions. Accessed April 2, 2019.

37. U.S. Preventive Services Task Force. Appendix I. Congressional mandate establishing the U.S. preventive services task force. Available at: https://www.uspreventiveservicestaskforce.org/Page/Name/appendix-i-congressional-mandate-establishing-the-us-preventive-services-task-force. Accessed April 2, 2019.

38. Huang YA, Zhu W, Smith DK, et al. HIV preexposure prophylaxis, by race and ethnicity—United States, 2014–2016. MMWR Morb Mortal Wkly Rep 2018;67: 1147–50. Available at: https://www.cdc.gov/mmwr/volumes/67/wr/mm6741a3.htm?s_cid=mm6741a3_w. Accessed April 3, 2019.

39. Marcus JL, Hurley LB, Hare CB, et al. Disparities in uptake of HIV preexposure prophylaxis in a large integrated health care system. Am J Public Health 2016;106:e2–3.

40. Marcus JL, Hurley LB, Dentoni-Lasofsky D, et al. Barriers to preexposure prophylaxis use among individuals with recently acquired HIV infection in Northern California. AIDS Care 2019;31:536–44.

41. Cahill S, Taylor SW, Elsesser SA, et al. Stigma, medical mistrust, and perceived racism may affect PrEP awareness and uptake in black compared to white gay and bisexual men in Jackson, Mississippi and Boston, Massachusetts. AIDS Care 2017;29:1351–8.

42. Rael CT, Martinez M, Giguere R, et al. Barriers and facilitators to oral PrEP use among transgender women in New York City. AIDS Behav 2018;22:3627–36.

43. Rowniak S, Ong-Flaherty C, Selix N, et al. Attitudes, beliefs, and barriers to PrEP among trans men. AIDS Educ Prev 2017;29:302–14.

44. Luthra S, Gorman A. Rising cost of PrEP to prevent HIV infection pushes it out of reach for many. NPR. 2018. Available at: https://www.npr.org/sections/health-shots/2018/06/30/624045995/rising-cost-of-prep-a-pill-that-prevents-hiv-pushes-it-out-of-reach-for-many. Accessed April 3, 2019.

45. Patel RR, Mena L, Nunn A, et al. Impact of insurance coverage on utilization of pre-exposure prophylaxis for HIV prevention. PLoS One 2017;12: e0178737.

46. Gilead. How can you get help paying for Truvada for PrEP?. Available at: https://www.truvada.com/how-to-get-truvada-for-prep/truvada-cost. Accessed April 3, 2019.

47. Petroll AE, Walsh JL, Owczarzak JL. PrEP awareness, familiarity, comfort, and prescribing experience among US primary care providers and HIV specialists. AIDS Behav 2017;21:1256–67.

48. Blackstock OJ, Moore BA, Berkenblit GV, et al. A cross-sectional online survey of HIV pre-exposure prophylaxis adoption among primary care physicians. J Gen Intern Med 2017;32(1): 62–70.

49. Silapaswan A, Krakower D, Mayer KH. Pre-exposure prophylaxis: a narrative review of provider behavior and interventions to increase PrEP implementation in primary care. J Gen Intern Med 2017; 32(2):192–8.

50. Chou R, Evans C, Hoverman A, et al. Pre-exposure prophylaxis for the prevention of HIV infection: a systematic review for the U.S. preventive services task force. Evidence synthesis no. 178. AHRQ Publication No. 18-05247-EF-1. Rockville (MD): Agency for Healthcare Research and Quality; 2018.

51. CDC. Comprehensive PrEP provider directory and locator. Available at: https://npin.cdc.gov/preplocator. Accessed April 3, 2019.

Androgenetic Alopecia in Gender Minority Patients

Dustin H. Marks, BS[a], Maryanne M. Senna, MD[a,b],*

KEYWORDS

- Gender minority • Transgender • Estrogen • Testosterone • Gender affirming hormone
- Androgenetic alopecia • Pattern hair loss • Minoxidil

KEY POINTS

- Hair represents an essential element of gender expression and perception.
- Androgens are a principal regulator of the hair cycle, whereas the role of estrogen is less clear and likely more complex.
- Moderate to severe androgenetic alopecia is less prevalent in transmen in comparison with similarly aged cismen.
- The clinical presentation of androgenetic alopecia as "male pattern" or "female pattern" may not match the gender identity of the patient.
- Minoxidil, low-level laser light therapy, and finasteride represent first-line treatments for androgenetic alopecia in gender minority patients.

INTRODUCTION

Androgenetic alopecia (AGA), also known as pattern hair loss, represents the most common subtype of hair loss, affecting 50% of individuals aged 40 years and older. This form of nonscarring alopecia involves a reduction in scalp hair density due to miniaturization of coarse terminal hairs to vellus hairs and prolongation of the telogen phase of the hair cycle.[1] Clinically, AGA occurs in 2 classic sex-based patterns, "male pattern" characterized by M-shaped recession of the frontal hairline and vertex thinning and "female pattern" involving a Christmas-tree thinning pattern disproportionally affecting the crown scalp. Although these distinct patterns may occur more frequently in each sex respectively, patients with AGA may display either pattern or a combination of both.[1,2]

Furthermore, the different clinical patterns of AGA may result from overlapping yet distinct etiologies. In cisgender men, AGA is androgen-dependent (eg, without androgens, AGA will not occur) and involves a predominant, polymorphic genetic predisposition.[3–5] Although androgen-related mechanisms and genetic predisposition likely contribute to the etiology of AGA in cisgender women, the pathogenesis remains more complex and accordingly, susceptibility loci have not been consistently identified.[5–7]

Although some clinicians may consider AGA to be a purely cosmetic issue, it can significantly affect an individual's self-image, social interactions, and overall quality of life.[2,8] Hair, moreover, remains a symbol of cultural, sexual, and religious persona, shaping an individual's identity, intimate relationships, social class, and work roles.[2,9] In addition, hair represents an essential element of gender expression and perception.[10,11] In accord, patients with AGA report high levels of stress and negative body image related to their hair loss, especially among cisgender women.[8,12,13]

Although the literature is limited, AGA may be particularly distressing for gender minority patients, given the close relation of hair to gender expression.[10] For transgender men, some may

a Department of Dermatology, Massachusetts General Hospital, 50 Staniford Street, Suite 200, Boston, MA 02114, USA; b Harvard Medical School, Boston, MA, USA
* Corresponding author. 50 Staniford Street, Suite 200, Boston, MA 02114.
E-mail address: msenna@partners.org

Dermatol Clin 38 (2020) 239–247
https://doi.org/10.1016/j.det.2019.10.010
0733-8635/20/© 2019 Elsevier Inc. All rights reserved.

embrace AGA as a desirable masculine trait, whereas others may seek treatment similar to some cisgender men.[14] For transgender women, AGA may be especially concerning, as hair loss, particularly with frontal M-shaped hairline recession and vertex thinning, represents a characteristically male phenotype. It is therefore critical that dermatologists are able to diagnose and treat AGA in gender minorities. In this review, we aim to summarize the role of gender affirming hormones on the hair cycle and discuss diagnosis and management of AGA in gender minority patients.

TERMINOLOGY

Gender identity reflects an individual's internal sense of being male, female, both, neither, or another gender. *Gender expression* is the outward display of gender, represented by an individual's clothing, hairstyle, speech, and mannerisms. *Transgender* accordingly serves as the umbrella term for individuals whose gender identity or gender expression differs from the sex that they were assigned at birth, typically based on external genital anatomy. More specifically, a *transgender woman* (or *transwoman*) is an individual who identifies as a woman with an assigned sex of male at birth. A *transgender man* (or *transman*) is an individual who identifies as a man with an assigned sex of female at birth. In addition, some individuals may identify with a gender that is more complex, fluid, or separate than the traditional dichotomous gender paradigm and may consider themselves as *gender nonconforming*, *nonbinary*, or *genderqueer*.[15] *Cisgender*, in contrast, references any individual who identifies with their sex assigned at birth (ie, an individual who identifies as a woman who was assigned the sex of female at birth).

EFFECT OF GENDER AFFIRMING HORMONES ON THE HAIR CYCLE

Use of gender affirming hormones, including testosterone in transmen and estrogen and antiandrogens in transwomen, has a direct impact on the hair growth cycle and ultimately leads to a change in the distribution and pattern of hair growth and density.[10]

Androgens

Androgens represent the principal regulator of the human hair cycle and demonstrate paradoxic effects on hair growth depending on the anatomic location.[16] These sex hormones bind to androgen receptors primarily at the level of the dermal papilla in addition to sebaceous glands and are converted into dihydrotestosterone (DHT; ie, the most potent human testosterone) by 5α-reductase.[17] Androgens can subsequently alter hair diameter, growth rate, length, and pigmentation. Whether the androgens ultimately stimulate hair to become longer/thicker/darker or shorter/finer/lighter depends on intrinsic gene expression that is determined by familial predisposition, sex, and body location.[16] In accord, androgen receptor sensitivity and distribution are region-specific, stimulating hair growth on the face, chest, axilla, and upper pubic diamond in contrast to hair loss on the scalp. This effect is best demonstrated in XY individuals with complete androgen insensitivity, who neither grow pubic/axillary hair nor develop AGA throughout their life course.[16,18]

Circulating levels of androgens and sensitivity/distribution of androgen receptors are relevant to hair growth and loss patterns.[19] In cisgender female individuals, normal levels of circulating androgens are sufficient to affect axillary and pubic follicles but typically do not affect facial follicles.[10,16,20] In cisgender male individuals, follicles on the mustache and chin regions are more androgen-sensitive than those on the lateral cheeks and neck.[21] In addition, frontal hairline follicles remain more androgen-sensitive than occipital follicles due to differences in 5α-reductase expression. Although androgens are further required for the development of AGA in cisgender men, they are generally not considered a prerequisite for AGA pathogenesis in cisgender women.[22,23]

Estrogens

In contrast to androgens, the effect of estrogen on the hair growth cycle is less clear and likely more intricate.[10] It is known that the pilosebaceous unit contains both aromatase and 17β-hydroxysteroid dehydrogenase, which are essential enzymes for the conversion of androgens to estrogen, and has a wide distribution of estrogen receptor beta (ERβ), implicating estrogen in the hair growth cycle.[20] Estrogen not only alters the transcription of genes directly related with estrogen-responsive elements but also modifies androgen metabolism, reducing levels of DHT.[10,20,24]

Current clinical and murine evidence, however, demonstrates an overall conflicting effect of estrogen on the hair cycle. On one hand, estrogens seem to prolong the anagen phase of the hair cycle, associated with overall increased hair density observed in pregnant and premenopausal women in comparison with nonpregnant and postmenopausal women, respectively.[10,25–27] In contrast, ex vivo murine models have shown that topical and parenteral estrogen antagonists are associated with significant hair growth, whereas estrogen agonists inhibit hair growth via telogen arrest.[10,22,28] The potential inhibitory effects of estrogen have been further supported in humans, as a specific allele for the aromatase-encoding gene associated with higher circulating estrogen levels was observed more frequently in cisgender women with AGA.[29] Further studies are thus critical to better understand the complex effect of estrogen on the hair cycle.

PREVALENCE OF ANDROGENETIC ALOPECIA IN GENDER MINORITIES

Although AGA is known to impact 50% of adults aged 40 and older, the exact prevalence rate of AGA in gender minorities is not known. Most of the existing evidence is limited to small sample sizes, almost exclusively focusing on European transmen on testosterone therapy. Recognizing these limitations, in a prospective study of 20 transmen (mean age 27 years), 1 (5%) patient developed mild frontotemporal hairline recession (Hamilton-Norwood II) after 1 year of intramuscular testosterone undecanoate (1000 mg) every 3 months.[30] In comparison, another 1-year prospective study found that 9 (17%) of 53 transmen (mean age 25 years) on the same testosterone regimen developed at least mild AGA.[31]

Another cross-sectional study assessed 50 transmen (mean age 37 years old) who had received a variety of testosterone therapies for an average of 10 years. Most (63.3%) transmen in this cohort demonstrated some degree of AGA, including 16 participants (32.7%) with only frontotemporal hairline recession (Hamilton-Norwood II) and 15 participants (31.0%) with moderate to severe AGA (Hamilton-Norwood III or above). Although no association was found with AGA and duration or subtype of testosterone therapy, there was a significant association with age (P = .03).[30] Of note, this study demonstrated a substantially lower prevalence of moderate to severe AGA in transmen aged 18 to 50 years old (25%) compared with a historic cohort of similarly aged cismen (42%).[30,32]

Moreover, there are several potential explanations for the lower prevalence of AGA in transmen. It is likely that an overall shorter duration of high-level testosterone exposure in transmen accounts for the lower prevalence of hair loss.[1,30] The higher average age at first exposure to high-level testosterone also may contribute to differences in AGA frequency. Alternatively, variances in levels of androgen receptors and steroid-converting enzymes could explain the lower rates of AGA in transmen. In a study of 24 cisgender patients, frontal hair follicles from ciswomen in comparison with cismen contained 40% less androgen receptor content, threefold less 5α-reductase, and sixfold more aromatase.[19] It is therefore possible that individuals assigned female at birth (AFAB) remain less likely to develop AGA. Nonetheless, these differences may change after long-term testosterone exposure, which could permanently alter gene expression at the level of the hair follicle.[16,30]

Recognizing that the overall prevalence of AGA may be lower in transmen than cismen, genetic predisposition remains an important factor to consider when assessing the potential risk of AGA development in transmen. In a therapeutic intervention study of 10 transmen with a mean onset of AGA being 3.25 years after initiation of testosterone treatment, 70% of patients reported a family history of AGA. Interestingly, transmen with a family history of AGA reported an earlier onset of hair loss (2.85 years after testosterone initiation) than transmen with no relevant family history (4.1 years after testosterone initiation).[14] In general, transmen may start to develop AGA 2 to 5 years after initiating testosterone therapy and the ultimate severity is likely dependent on age and genetic predisposition.[10,33]

In comparison with transmen, there are effectively no data on the prevalence of AGA in transwomen and gender nonbinary patients. Based on the natural course of AGA in individuals assigned male at birth, transwomen who initiate estrogen and antiandrogen therapy at a later age (eg, fifth or sixth decade of life) may be more likely to develop frontal M-shaped recession of the hairline and vertex thinning than transwomen who start gender affirming hormones at an earlier age (eg, second or third decade of life).[1] This postulation, though, has not been studied to date.

DIAGNOSIS OF ANDROGENETIC ALOPECIA IN GENDER MINORITIES

A similar approach to the evaluation and diagnosis of hair loss in the general adult population can be applied to diagnosing AGA in gender minority patients with several nuances to consider.[1,34] A thorough history remains a vital tool for the development of a differential diagnosis and is especially critical to rule out telogen effluvium (TE).[1] When eliciting TE risk factors in gender minority patients, it is important to explicitly ask about oral contraceptives and other hormonal forms of birth control, gender affirming hormones, pregnancy and childbirth, major surgeries including gender affirming surgeries, and increased emotional stress. Inquiring about the timeline of gender affirming treatments and procedures, if any, are particularly relevant, as changes in hormonal medications and major surgeries represent common TE risk factors.[35,36] Also of consideration, some transgender men and gender nonbinary patients retain their uterus and may become pregnant and give birth. Due to societal attitudes, they may be less likely to disclose relevant history around contraception and pregnancy unless directly asked.[37]

To supplement a detailed history, the clinical examination will aid in the diagnosis of AGA. It is important to note that the specific stereotyped AGA pattern (ie, "male pattern" as a receding hairline and vertex thinning vs "female pattern" as a wider midline part at the crown) may not match the gender identity of the patient and/or there may be considerable overlap of these typically distinct distributions in gender minority patients. To date, there have been no reported cases of classic "female-pattern" hair loss in transwomen, whereas there are numerous cases of "male-pattern" hair loss in transmen and transwomen.[10,14] For any given patient, nonetheless, the ultimate phenotype of AGA is likely multifactorial and dependent on sex assigned at birth; genetic predisposition; comorbid conditions (eg, polycystic ovary syndrome, diabetes, hypothyroidism); and exposure, age at first use, and duration of gender affirming hormones.[1,31,34,38]

In addition to an assessment of the hair loss pattern, a close examination of the scalp is critical to rule out a scarring (or cicatricial) form of hair loss.[34,39–41] Lichen planopilaris (LPP) and its variant frontal fibrosing alopecia (FFA) represent 2 of the more common forms of cicatricial alopecia, although relatively rare overall.[42] These conditions primarily affect postmenopausal white ciswomen, although their prevalence in gender minority patients is currently unknown.[43,44] Given this selective demographic, it is likely that environmental, genetic, and hormonal factors all contribute to the pathogenesis of LPP/FFA.[45,46] Supporting low estrogen as a potential risk factor for FFA, a case-control study of ciswomen found a positive association of FFA with early menopause/tamoxifen use and a negative association with intrauterine device use.[46] As use of testosterone in transmen significantly lowers estradiol levels, it may be associated with a theoretically increased risk of FFA development.[47] Although more research is necessary to establish this association, a close inspection of the scalp remains paramount to ruling out scarring hair loss before establishing an official diagnosis of AGA in gender minority patients.

TREATMENT OF ANDROGENETIC ALOPECIA IN GENDER MINORITIES

Despite the prevalence of AGA, the Food and Drug Administration (FDA) has approved only 3 medical treatments for this condition, including topical minoxidil and low-level laser light therapy (LLLLT) for both male- and female-pattern hair loss and oral finasteride for male-pattern hair loss. This section is meant to emphasize special considerations of FDA-approved therapeutic modalities in gender minority patients.

Nonhormonal Treatments

Minoxidil and LLLLT represent 2 effective and safe treatments for AGA in gender minority patients and have no known interactions with gender affirming hormones.

Minoxidil

Initially developed for refractory hypertension, minoxidil represents one of the most extensively researched and effective treatments for AGA. Although the exact mechanism is unknown, this medication may promote hair growth by lengthening the anagen phase, shortening the telogen phase, and enlarging miniaturized hair follicles.[48,49] Its vasodilator properties may also help to increase vascularity and the size of dermal papillae.[50,51]

Currently, 5% minoxidil foam or solution twice daily is recommended for men, whereas 5% foam once daily or 2% solution twice daily is recommend for women.[10,48,52] To date, no study has investigated the dosing schedule of minoxidil in gender minority patients. Clinicians may consider starting 5% minoxidil foam twice daily in gender minority patients (given the frequency of "male pattern" in both transmen and transwomen) and decreasing if scalp irritation develops. The most common side effects are contact dermatitis and facial hypertrichosis, which occur more commonly in higher concentration formulations.[48,53,54] Interestingly, hypertrichosis is reported more frequently in ciswomen than cismen, but it is not known if this is a true variance or simply more noticeable or bothersome.[48]

For patients with moderate to severe AGA, low-dose oral minoxidil may represent another effective treatment. In a prospective cohort study, 100 ciswomen with AGA were treated with oral minoxidil 0.25 mg and spironolactone 25 mg for 1 year. There was a significant mean reduction in hair loss severity score (1.3 on the Sinclair Scale) and hair shedding score. The regimen was well tolerated with only 8 patients reporting adverse events, including postural hypotension, hypertrichosis, and urticaria.[55] Although it is not currently commercially available, low-dose oral minoxidil is an important treatment option for AGA in gender minorities, as it represents one of the only systemic medications that does not have hormonal properties or interact with gender affirming hormones. In addition, the adverse event of hypertrichosis may be desirable to some transmen and genderqueer patients.

Low-level laser light therapy

Representing the most recent FDA-approved treatment for AGA, LLLLT has demonstrated utility for hair regrowth in double-blind, sham device-controlled trials.[56,57] It is postulated that LLLLT stimulates hair follicle stem cells and may also have anti-inflammatory properties.[58–61] In a multicenter, randomized control trial of 110 men with AGA, those who used a handheld LLLLT (655 nm) for 15 minutes 3 times per week had a significantly greater increase in mean terminal hair density and improvement in subjective self-assessment of hair regrowth than control patients who used a sham device.[56] The efficacy of LLLLT for AGA has similarly been demonstrated in women.[57]

This therapy, furthermore, is very well tolerated, as patients report few and mild adverse events, including dryness, itching, and a warm sensation.[52] Accordingly, LLLLT serves as a safe and effective treatment intervention for AGA and, as an external device, has no known interactions with hormonal therapy. All patients, irrespective of sex or gender identity, will follow the same dosage recommendation for LLLLT: at least 3 times per week for a specific interval of time dependent on the model, which includes helmets, bands, combs, and wands.[62]

Hormonal Treatments

Antiandrogen therapies, such as finasteride and spironolactone, represent efficacious treatments for AGA. There are, however, several unique considerations for their use in gender minority patients. As 49% of gender minority patients are on hormone therapy, many transwomen and some gender nonbinary patients may already take finasteride and/or spironolactone.[63] In fact, reduced body/facial hair and increased scalp hair represent 2 major purposes for initiating feminizing hormone therapy in general.[33,64] Nonetheless, the degree of hair regrowth and utility of these medications as monotherapies for AGA in transwomen is unknown. Several case reports have suggested substantial hair regrowth in transwomen treated with hormone therapies but the evidence is limited.[65,66]

In transmen and other gender minority patients on testosterone, use of antiandrogen therapies should be recommended with caution, as they may interfere with the development of desired secondary sex characteristics (eg, deepened voice, increased body hair, clitoromegaly). As most physical changes occur within the first 2 years of hormone therapy, finasteride or spironolactone should not be started until at least that time.[67] However, some changes such as increased muscle mass/strength and body fat redistribution may take up to 5 years to completely develop and thus with a more conservative approach, some patients may opt to start antiandrogen therapy after at least 5 years of testosterone.[33] In addition, it is critical that clinicians discuss the teratogenic effects of these medications with transmen and other individuals AFAB, who may retain the ability to become pregnant.

Finasteride

Finasteride represents one of the most effective treatments for AGA in cismen but has demonstrated more equivocal results in ciswomen.[68–70] It functions as a competitive inhibitor of 5α-reductase, lowering scalp and serum DHT levels by 64.1% and 71.4%, respectively, at oral dosages of 1 mg daily in cismen.[71] To date, only 1 small prospective cohort study has investigated the use of finasteride in transmen.[14] More specifically, 10 transmen (mean age 35 years) with a baseline severity of stage IV on the Hamilton-Norwood scale were followed for at least 1 year on oral finasteride 1 mg daily. All patients improved at least 1 severity grade and no sexual or physical changes were noted, although 3 patients discontinued due to financial burden or dyspepsia. Ultimately, the investigators concluded that "male-pattern" AGA in transmen is clinically and therapeutically similar to "male-pattern" AGA in cismen and can be effectively treated with oral finasteride 1 mg daily.[14]

Although the evidence is limited by the small study sample, oral finasteride 1 mg daily can be recommended for AGA in transmen after at least 2 years on testosterone therapy. However, its efficacy for AGA in transwomen is unknown. If transwomen display frontal M-shaped hairline recession with vertex thinning that developed before the initiation of hormone therapy, oral finasteride 1 mg daily may be beneficial for hair regrowth.

For gender minority patients, a relevant and tailored discussion of the safety profile of finasteride may be dependent on his/her/their prior gender affirming surgeries, and it is therefore critical that clinicians inquire about surgical history appropriately. Relevant adverse events may include but are not limited to the teratogenic properties, sexual side effects (eg, decreased libido, erectile dysfunction), gynecomastia, and reduced prostate-specific antigen serum levels.[48,72–74] Also of concern, depression and suicidal ideation (predominantly in the context of permanent sexual dysfunction) have been reported in association with finasteride use.[48,75,76] As there are high rates of depression, and suicidal ideation and attempt among gender minorities, these potential risk factors of finasteride should be routinely discussed, recognizing that AGA also is associated with reduced quality of life and depression.[8,48,77,78]

Given these potential risk factors and interference with testosterone therapy, topical finasteride may represent an attractive treatment for AGA in gender minority patients. A recent systematic review concluded that use of topical finasteride is a safe and effective intervention with potentially fewer long-term side effects than oral finasteride.[79] However, a topical solution of 0.25% finasteride with 3% minoxidil was associated with significantly reduced plasma DHT levels by 5% in cismen and 33% in ciswomen.[80,81] These values, though, are substantially less than the 71.4% reduction in serum DHT seen with oral finasteride 1 mg daily.[71] In addition, topical finasteride is currently not commercially available in the United States and requires a compounding pharmacy, averaging a higher monthly expense than the oral version.

Hair Transplantation

For the best long-term results, hair transplantation should be performed in patients with medically controlled, stabilized AGA for at least 2 years to reduce postoperative progression.[52] To date, only one study has investigated hair transplantation with simultaneous forehead reconstruction in 65 transwomen (mean age 38 years).[82] Capitán and colleagues[82] described a surgical technique involving reconstruction of the fronto-naso-orbital complex in addition to a simultaneous follicular unit strip surgery to the frontal hairline. Due to the potential adverse events of a visible scar line and excessively short forehead, the investigators advocate for autologous hair transplantation as opposed to hairline-lowering surgery in transwomen. In addition, given the frequency of forehead reconstruction in transwomen who also seek hairline correction, these procedures may be simplified with a more successful outcome when performed concurrently.[82]

MANAGEMENT OF ANDROGENETIC ALOPECIA IN GENDER MINORITIES

As with all patients, setting realistic expectations about hair regrowth and obtaining consistent assessment measures is critical. Regardless of the specific treatment modality, topical, laser, and oral interventions should be continued for at least 6 to 12 months before the degree of hair regrowth is evaluated and continued indefinitely to sustain benefit. To assess initial severity and track progression, a number of AGA classification systems have been proposed, although most are sex-specific.[83] For gender minority patients, more general, non–sex-based scales (eg, Bouhanna or Basic and Specific Classification) may be used.[84,85] Alternatively, "male-pattern" and "female-pattern" specific scales, such as the Hamilton-Norwood and Sinclair scales, respectively, can be used in conjunction for AGA assessment.[86,87] Global photography also represents an effective, semiobjective, non–sex-specific tool in hair growth evaluation.[52]

SUMMARY

As hair represents an essential element of gender expression, AGA may be particularly distressing to gender minority patients and in particular, transwomen. Although a similar approach to diagnosing and treating AGA in cisgender patients can be applied to gender minority patients, there are several critical differences to consider with regard to pertinent TE risk factors, hair loss pattern, and treatment counseling. Ultimately, clinicians should recognize the impact of gender affirming hormones on the hair growth cycle and comfortably treat androgenetic alopecia in all patients regardless of gender identity.

DISCLOSURE

The authors have no commercial or financial conflicts of interest to disclose. This article had no funding sources.

REFERENCES

1. Otberg N, Shapiro J. Chapter 88. Hair growth disorders. In: Goldsmith LA, Katz SI, Gilchrest BA, et al, editors. Fitzpatrick's dermatology in general medicine, 8e | AccessMedicine | McGraw-Hill Medical. 8th edition. New York: The McGraw-Hill Companies; 2012. Available at: https://accessmedicine-mhmedical-com.ezp-prod1.hul.harvard.edu/Content.aspx?bookId=392&sectionId=41138795. Accessed September 6, 2018.

2. Olsen EA, editor. Disorders of hair growth: diagnosis and treatment. 2nd edition. New York: McGraw-Hill, Medical Pub. Division; 2003.

3. Hamilton JB. Male hormone stimulation is prerequisite and an incitant in common baldness. Am J Anat 1942;71(3):451–80.

4. Ellis JA, Stebbing M, Harrap SB. Genetic analysis of male pattern baldness and the 5alpha-reductase genes. J Invest Dermatol 1998;110(6):849–53.

5. Redler S, Messenger AG, Betz RC. Genetics and other factors in the aetiology of female pattern hair loss. Exp Dermatol 2017;26(6):510–7.

6. Redler S, Brockschmidt FF, Tazi-Ahnini R, et al. Investigation of the male pattern baldness major genetic susceptibility loci AR/EDA2R and 20p11 in female pattern hair loss. Br J Dermatol 2012;166(6):1314–8.

7. Nuwaihyd R, Redler S, Heilmann S, et al. Investigation of four novel male androgenetic alopecia susceptibility loci: no association with female pattern hair loss. Arch Dermatol Res 2014;306(4):413–8.

8. Marks DH, Penzi LR, Ibler E, et al. The medical and psychosocial associations of alopecia: recognizing hair loss as more than a cosmetic concern. Am J Clin Dermatol 2018. https://doi.org/10.1007/s40257-018-0405-2.

9. Weitz R. Rapunzel's daughters: what women's hair tells us about women's lives. New York: Macmillan; 2004.

10. Gao Y, Maurer T, Mirmirani P. Understanding and addressing hair disorders in transgender individuals. Am J Clin Dermatol 2018;19(4):517–27.

11. Synnott A. Shame and glory: a sociology of hair. Br J Sociol 1987;38(3):381–413.

12. van der Donk J, Passchier J, Knegt-Junk C, et al. Psychological characteristics of women with androgenetic alopecia: a controlled study. Br J Dermatol 1991;125(3):248–52.

13. Cash TF. The psychosocial consequences of androgenetic alopecia: a review of the research literature. Br J Dermatol 1999;141(3):398–405.

14. Moreno-Arrones OM, Becerra A, Vano-Galvan S. Therapeutic experience with oral finasteride for androgenetic alopecia in female-to-male transgender patients. Clin Exp Dermatol 2017;42(7):743–8.

15. Deutsch M. Guidelines for the primary and gender-affirming care of transgender and gender nonbinary people: introduction to the guidelines. San Francisco, CA: Center of Excellence for Transgender Health; 2016. Available at: http://transhealth.ucsf.edu/pdf/Transgender-PGACG-6-17-16.pdf. Accessed September 17, 2018.

16. Randall VA. Androgens and hair growth. Dermatol Ther 2008;21(5):314–28.

17. Itami S, Inui S. Role of androgen in mesenchymal epithelial interactions in human hair follicle. J Investig Dermatol Symp Proc 2005;10(3):209–11.

18. Hughes IA, Davies JD, Bunch TI, et al. Androgen insensitivity syndrome. Lancet 2012;380(9851):1419–28.

19. Sawaya ME, Price VH. Different levels of 5alpha-reductase type I and II, aromatase, and androgen receptor in hair follicles of women and men with androgenetic alopecia. J Invest Dermatol 1997;109(3):296–300.

20. Ohnemus U, Uenalan M, Inzunza J, et al. The hair follicle as an estrogen target and source. Endocr Rev 2006;27(6):677–706.

21. Marshall WA, Tanner JM. Variations in the pattern of pubertal changes in boys. Arch Dis Child 1970;45(239):13–23.

22. Yip L, Rufaut N, Sinclair R. Role of genetics and sex steroid hormones in male androgenetic alopecia and female pattern hair loss: an update of what we now know: update on androgenetic alopecia. Australas J Dermatol 2011;52(2):81–8.

23. Olsen EA, Messenger AG, Shapiro J, et al. Evaluation and treatment of male and female pattern hair loss. J Am Acad Dermatol 2005;52(2):301–11.

24. Niiyama S, Happle R, Hoffmann R. Influence of estrogens on the androgen metabolism in different subunits of human hair follicles. Eur J Dermatol 2001;11(3):195–8.

25. Schumacher JR, Taylor LJ, Tucholka JL, et al. Socioeconomic factors associated with post-mastectomy immediate reconstruction in a contemporary cohort of breast cancer survivors. Ann Surg Oncol 2017;24(10):3017–23.

26. Nelson LR, Bulun SE. Estrogen production and action. J Am Acad Dermatol 2001;45(3, Supplement):S116–24.

27. Lynfield YL. Effect of pregnancy on the human hair cycle. J Invest Dermatol 1960;35:323–7.

28. Oh HS, Smart RC. An estrogen receptor pathway regulates the telogen-anagen hair follicle transition and influences epidermal cell proliferation. Proc Natl Acad Sci U S A 1996;93(22):12525–30.

29. Yip L, Zaloumis S, Irwin D, et al. Gene-wide association study between the aromatase gene (CYP19A1) and female pattern hair loss. Br J Dermatol 2009;161(2):289–94.

30. Wierckx K, Van de Peer F, Verhaeghe E, et al. Short- and long-term clinical skin effects of testosterone treatment in trans men. J Sex Med 2014;11(1):222–9.

31. Wierckx K, Van Caenegem E, Schreiner T, et al. Cross-sex hormone therapy in trans persons is safe and effective at short-time follow-up: results from the european network for the investigation of gender incongruence. J Sex Med 2014;11(8):1999–2011.

32. Rhodes T, Girman CJ, Savin RC, et al. Prevalence of male pattern hair loss in 18-49 year old men. Dermatol Surg 1998;24(12):1330–2.

33. Coleman E, Bockting W, Botzer M, et al. Standards of care for the health of transsexual, transgender, and gender-nonconforming people, version 7. Int J Transgend 2012;13(4):165–232.

34. Mubki T, Rudnicka L, Olszewska M, et al. Evaluation and diagnosis of the hair loss patient: part I. History and clinical examination. J Am Acad Dermatol 2014; 71(3):415.e1-15.

35. Malkud S. Telogen effluvium: a review. J Clin Diagn Res 2015;9(9):WE01–3.

36. Headington JT. Telogen effluvium: new concepts and review. Arch Dermatol 1993;129(3):356–63.

37. Hoffkling A, Obedin-Maliver J, Sevelius J. From erasure to opportunity: a qualitative study of the experiences of transgender men around pregnancy and recommendations for providers. BMC Pregnancy Childbirth 2017;17(Suppl 2). https://doi.org/ 10.1186/s12884-017-1491-5.

38. Shapiro J. Hair loss in women. N Engl J Med 2007; 357(16):1620–30.

39. Filbrandt R, Rufaut N, Jones L, et al. Primary cicatricial alopecia: diagnosis and treatment. Can Med Assoc J 2013;185(18):1579–85.

40. Shapiro J. Cicatricial alopecias. Dermatol Ther 2008; 21(4):211.

41. Harries MJ, Trueb RM, Tosti A, et al. How not to get scar(r)ed: pointers to the correct diagnosis in patients with suspected primary cicatricial alopecia. Br J Dermatol 2009;160(3):482–501.

42. Ochoa BE, King LE, Price VH. Lichen planopilaris: annual incidence in four hair referral centers in the United States. J Am Acad Dermatol 2008;58(2): 352–3.

43. Kossard S. Postmenopausal frontal fibrosing alopecia. Scarring alopecia in a pattern distribution. Arch Dermatol 1994;130(6):770–4.

44. Tan E, Martinka M, Ball N, et al. Primary cicatricial alopecias: clinicopathology of 112 cases. J Am Acad Dermatol 2004;50(1):25–32.

45. Aldoori N, Dobson K, Holden CR, et al. Frontal fibrosing alopecia: possible association with leave-on facial skin care products and sunscreens; a questionnaire study. Br J Dermatol 2016;175(4):762–7.

46. Buendía-Castaño D, Saceda-Corralo D, Moreno-Arrones OM, et al. Hormonal and gynecological risk factors in frontal fibrosing alopecia: a case-control study. Skin Appendage Disord 2018;4(4): 274–6.

47. Chan KJ, Jolly D, Liang JJ, et al. Estrogen levels do not rise with testosterone treatment for transgender men. Endocr Pract 2018;24(4):329–33.

48. Kelly Y, Blanco A, Tosti A. Androgenetic alopecia: an update of treatment options. Drugs 2016;76(14): 1349–64.

49. Messenger AG, Rundegren J. Minoxidil: mechanisms of action on hair growth. Br J Dermatol 2004;150(2):186–94.

50. Lachgar S, Charveron M, Gall Y, et al. Minoxidil up-regulates the expression of vascular endothelial growth factor in human hair dermal papilla cells. Br J Dermatol 1998;138(3):407–11.

51. Li M, Marubayashi A, Nakaya Y, et al. Minoxidil-induced hair growth is mediated by adenosine in cultured dermal papilla cells: possible involvement of sulfonylurea receptor 2B as a target of minoxidil. J Invest Dermatol 2001;117(6):1594–600.

52. Kanti V, Messenger A, Dobos G, et al. Evidence-based (S3) guideline for the treatment of androgenetic alopecia in women and in men – short version. J Eur Acad Dermatol Venereol 2018;32(1):11–22.

53. Dawber RPR, Rundegren J. Hypertrichosis in females applying minoxidil topical solution and in normal controls. J Eur Acad Dermatol Venereol 2003;17(3):271–5.

54. Lucky AW, Piacquadio DJ, Ditre CM, et al. A randomized, placebo-controlled trial of 5% and 2% topical minoxidil solutions in the treatment of female pattern hair loss. J Am Acad Dermatol 2004; 50(4):541–53.

55. Sinclair RD. Female pattern hair loss: a pilot study investigating combination therapy with low-dose oral minoxidil and spironolactone. Int J Dermatol 2018;57(1):104–9.

56. Leavitt M, Charles G, Heyman E, et al. HairMax LaserComb laser phototherapy device in the treatment of male androgenetic alopecia: a randomized, double-blind, sham device-controlled, multicentre trial. Clin Drug Investig 2009;29(5):283–92.

57. Jimenez JJ, Wikramanayake TC, Bergfeld W, et al. Efficacy and safety of a low-level laser device in the treatment of male and female pattern hair loss: a multicenter, randomized, sham device-controlled, double-blind study. Am J Clin Dermatol 2014;15(2): 115–27.

58. Eells JT, Wong-Riley MTT, VerHoeve J, et al. Mitochondrial signal transduction in accelerated wound and retinal healing by near-infrared light therapy. Mitochondrion 2004;4(5–6):559–67.

59. Pastore D, Greco M, Passarella S. Specific helium-neon laser sensitivity of the purified cytochrome c oxidase. Int J Radiat Biol 2000;76(6):863–70.

60. Arany PR, Nayak RS, Hallikerimath S, et al. Activation of latent TGF-beta1 by low-power laser in vitro correlates with increased TGF-beta1 levels in laser-enhanced oral wound healing. Wound Repair Regen 2007;15(6):866–74.

61. Sakurai Y, Yamaguchi M, Abiko Y. Inhibitory effect of low-level laser irradiation on LPS-stimulated prostaglandin E2 production and cyclooxygenase-2 in human gingival fibroblasts. Eur J Oral Sci 2000;108(1): 29–34.

62. Frequently asked questions. HairMax. Available at: https://hairmax.com/pages/faq-1. Accessed November 14, 2019.

63. James SE, Herman JL, Rankin S, et al. The report of the 2015 U.S. transgender survey. Washington, DC: National Center for Transgender Equality; 2016.

64. Unger CA. Hormone therapy for transgender patients. Transl Androl Urol 2016;5(6):877–84.

65. Stevenson MO, Wixon N, Safer JD. Scalp hair regrowth in hormone-treated transgender woman. Transgend Health 2016;1(1):202–4.

66. Adenuga P, Summers P, Bergfeld W. Hair regrowth in a male patient with extensive androgenetic alopecia on estrogen therapy. J Am Acad Dermatol 2012; 67(3):e121–3.

67. Ginsberg BA. Dermatologic care of the transgender patient. Int J Womens Dermatol 2016;3(1):65–7.

68. Adil A, Godwin M. The effectiveness of treatments for androgenetic alopecia: a systematic review and meta-analysis. J Am Acad Dermatol 2017;77(1): 136–41.e5.

69. Price VH, Roberts JL, Hordinsky M, et al. Lack of efficacy of finasteride in postmenopausal women with androgenetic alopecia. J Am Acad Dermatol 2000; 43(5 Pt 1):768–76.

70. Carmina E, Lobo RA. Treatment of hyperandrogenic alopecia in women. Fertil Steril 2003;79(1):91–5.

71. Drake L, Hordinsky M, Fiedler V, et al. The effects of finasteride on scalp skin and serum androgen levels in men with androgenetic alopecia. J Am Acad Dermatol 1999;41(4):550–4.

72. Mella JM, Perret MC, Manzotti M, et al. Efficacy and safety of finasteride therapy for androgenetic alopecia: a systematic review. Arch Dermatol 2010; 146(10):1141–50.

73. Mansouri P, Farshi S, Safar F. Finasteride-induced gynecomastia. Indian J Dermatol Venereol Leprol 2009;75(3):309–10.

74. D'Amico AV, Roehrborn CG. Effect of 1 mg/day finasteride on concentrations of serum prostate-specific antigen in men with androgenic alopecia: a randomised controlled trial. Lancet Oncol 2007; 8(1):21–5.

75. Ali AK, Heran BS, Etminan M. Persistent sexual dysfunction and suicidal ideation in young men treated with low-dose finasteride: a pharmacovigilance study. Pharmacotherapy 2015;35(7):687–95.

76. Irwig MS. Depressive symptoms and suicidal thoughts among former users of finasteride with persistent sexual side effects. J Clin Psychiatry 2012;73(9):1220–3.

77. Clements-Nolle K, Marx R, Guzman R, et al. HIV prevalence, risk behaviors, health care use, and mental health status of transgender persons: implications for public health intervention. Am J Public Health 2001;91(6):915–21.

78. Clements-Nolle K, Marx R, Katz M. Attempted suicide among transgender persons: the influence of gender-based discrimination and victimization. J Homosex 2006;51(3):53–69.

79. Lee SW, Juhasz M, Mobasher P, et al. A systematic review of topical finasteride in the treatment of androgenetic alopecia in men and women. J Drugs Dermatol 2018;17(4):457–63.

80. Suchonwanit P, Srisuwanwattana P, Chalermroj N, et al. A randomized, double-blind controlled study of the efficacy and safety of topical solution of 0.25% finasteride admixed with 3% minoxidil vs. 3% minoxidil solution in the treatment of male androgenetic alopecia. J Eur Acad Dermatol Venereol 2018;32(12):2257–63.

81. Suchonwanit P, Iamsumang W, Rojhirunsakool S. Efficacy of topical combination of 0.25% finasteride and 3% minoxidil versus 3% minoxidil solution in female pattern hair loss: a randomized, double-blind, controlled study. Am J Clin Dermatol 2019;20(1): 147–53.

82. Capitán L, Simon D, Meyer T, et al. Facial feminization surgery: simultaneous hair transplant during forehead reconstruction. Plast Reconstr Surg 2017; 139(3):573–84.

83. Gupta M, Mysore V. Classifications of patterned hair loss: a review. J Cutan Aesthet Surg 2016;9(1):3–12.

84. Bouhanna P. Multifactorial classification of male and female androgenetic alopecia. Dermatol Surg 2000; 26(6):555–61.

85. Lee W-S, Ro BI, Hong SP, et al. A new classification of pattern hair loss that is universal for men and women: basic and specific (BASP) classification. J Am Acad Dermatol 2007;57(1):37–46.

86. Norwood OT. Male pattern baldness: classification and incidence. South Med J 1975;68(11):1359–65.

87. Sinclair R, Jolley D, Mallari R, et al. The reliability of horizontally sectioned scalp biopsies in the diagnosis of chronic diffuse telogen hair loss in women. J Am Acad Dermatol 2004;51(2):189–99.

Minimally Invasive Procedures for Gender Affirmation

Jennifer L. MacGregor, MD*, Yunyoung C. Chang, MD

KEYWORDS

- Transgender • Nonbinary • Gender affirmation • Nonsurgical cosmetic procedures
- Minimally invasive cosmetic procedures • Noninvasive cosmetic procedures • Masculinization
- Feminization

KEY POINTS

- Although medical and surgical therapy may induce aesthetic transformations in the transgender population, the barriers to access and anatomic changes may be slower than desired, often taking months to years.
- With the growing number of transgender patients transitioning, dermatologists play an important role in improving outreach, implementing transgender-friendly practices, and formulating customized medical/cosmetic treatment plans.
- Dermatologists can address cosmetic concerns, including gender-affirming facial and body contouring, hormone-related skin changes, and surgery-related scarring.
- Aesthetic preferences may not follow the traditional binary ideals of beauty, including masculine versus feminine, and should be personalized during the initial consultation and subsequent follow-ups.
- Increased dermatologic literature detailing the available treatments for transgender transition and effects on quality of life is needed.

INTRODUCTION
Epidemiology of the Transgender Population

The reported overall prevalence of the transgender population has increased over the past decade, with 1 study reporting about 0.6% of adults (approximately 1.4 million) and 0.7% of youth aged 13 to 17 years (approximately 150,000 youth) identify as transgender in the United States.[1,2] This estimate is double those from prior studies less than a decade ago.[1,2] As the awareness and prevalence of the transgender population increases, it will be important to ensure that all health care providers are well versed in caring for this population.

Role of Dermatologists and Other Physicians

Dermatologists are starting to address practice gaps and consider a more supportive role in the care of their transgender patients.[3,4] Dermatologists play a critical role in both the medical and aesthetic care of transgender patients. Transgender patients present with similar dermatologic conditions as the general population as well as distinct cosmetic concerns during the transition process.[3] For example, acne is a common problem in transgender men undergoing testosterone therapy,[5] and recent dermatologic literature calls for a change from the current the gender-binary iPLEDGE labeling system for isotretinoin prescriptions to a more inclusive system that allows appropriate care of all gender orientations. In addition to general dermatologic concerns, cosmetic concerns are especially tied to the emotional well-being of transgender patients, because, by definition, their identity and desired aesthetic presentation to the world differ from their biological

Union Square Laser Dermatology, 19 Union Square West, 5th Floor, New York, NY 10003, USA
* Corresponding author.
E-mail address: jmacgregormd@gmail.com

Dermatol Clin 38 (2020) 249–260
https://doi.org/10.1016/j.det.2019.10.014

sex assigned at birth or chromosomal sex. Cosmetic concerns may include gender-affirming facial and body contouring, hormone-related skin changes, and surgery-related scarring.[3] It is also essential to consider that each patient's aesthetic goals may differ from the traditional masculine or feminine ideals of beauty as listed in **Box 1**.[6–8] This article instead advocates a more fluid result that is patient directed and suits each individual.

Physicians must also consider the many barriers transgender individuals face as they navigate their transition process in order to understand the reasons patients might consider care outside of traditional medicine.[9] Unlicensed providers, international Internet prescriptions, or illegal products are often used when patients seeking transition face barriers they think are insurmountable. Medical providers can themselves become a barrier to good care (often referred to in the community as

gatekeepers) because of their ability to decide, delay, and regulate prescriptions or aesthetic treatments that may not seem acceptable to the patients' timeline. Board-certified providers may also charge more money for procedures, and lack of insurance coverage for aesthetics make some of these treatments cost-prohibitive for patients without the necessary disposable income. Further, location far from metropolitan areas and lack of family or social support make access difficult for many. Faced with societal pressures to conform to masculine or feminine ideals of beauty but stopped by the barriers to receiving needed medical care or aesthetic procedures, transitioning patients may experience anxiety and depression. It is understandable, then, why some transgender patients resort to "pumping", or using liquid silicone,[10,11] or receive care from untrained, unqualified providers. The appropriate response of physicians in these cases is to meet the patients where they are, avoid condescending language regarding the patients' decisions, listen, and develop a plan to help move forward. The office staff and physicians must also be trained to ask and address patients with their preferred pronouns and ensure that office medical forms are inclusive of all gender orientations. With compassionate, supportive care and better marketing outreach, clinicians can bring more transgender patients into the care of board-certified and qualified physicians.

Noninvasive aesthetic procedures performed by board-certified physicians have clear advantages. Laser treatments and injectables are performed in an outpatient medical setting with high safety standards, minimal risk, and little downtime compared with surgery. Facial injectables are mostly reversible and can be started immediately to enhance, reduce, masculinize, or feminize features according to the patients' goals. There is minimal need for psychological vetting, pretreatment medication, or other delays that would be routinely needed before invasive surgery. In cisgender patients, minimally invasive aesthetic procedures have been shown to improve body image, self-esteem, and quality of life (QOL).[12]

Educational resources and published data are available regarding hormonal therapy and surgical procedures to support gender transition. However, the dermatologic literature on minimally invasive procedures is currently sparse. Specifics on how dermatologists can assist in the aesthetic transformation of transgender patients, meet their individual goals, and thereby improve QOL need to be elucidated. Current reviews[8,13] consolidate and outline current literature providing useful guides to providers, but new case series, before and after

---

Box 1
Selected traditional masculine versus feminine features

- Traditionally masculine features
  - Higher, possibly receding hairline
  - Wider, more angular forehead
  - Flat, horizontal brow
  - More prominent supraorbital brow ridges
  - Wider mouth with thinner lips
  - Longer, more square chin
  - Wider, more square lower face
  - Beard hair or coarser lower face skin texture
  - Acute nasolabial angle
- Traditionally feminine features
  - Lower hairline
  - Smooth, convex forehead
  - Brows arch above softer orbital rim
  - Eyes appear more open and/or wider set
  - Convex, prominent cheek contour
  - Heart-shaped, more tapered lower face
  - Smaller lower face to upper face proportion
  - Fuller vermillion contour and fuller lip body
  - More obtuse nasolabial angle

The authors instead advocate more fluid, patient-directed aesthetic goals that may not adhere to the following ideals.
Data from Refs.[6–8]

images, larger studies, and new data are needed. The authors think that all patients can benefit from noninvasive aesthetic procedures to support their aesthetic goals for their appearance and improve their outcomes when transitioning. Studies are underway to assess QOL data specifically in transgender individuals who have received noninvasive aesthetic dermatologic services to quantify the impact and improve future counseling efforts. This article reviews the common factors and medications affecting gender transition as well as the noninvasive cosmetic procedures as they relate specifically to the transgender population (including some case examples). Readers should keep an open mind that the aesthetic procedures transgender patients seek may be feminizing, masculinizing, both, or neither. Practitioners must ask patients about their goals, listen to all patients, and speak candidly about their preferences before proceeding with recommendations and treatments.

Overview: Medications and Procedures Available to Assist with Gender Transition

Transgender individuals may choose to transition socially, medically, and/or surgically to align their gender expressions with their gender identities.[14] Hormonal therapy has become more widely prescribed for the transgender population.[15] Medical guidelines have been created by the World Professional Association for Transgender Health and the Endocrine Society to guide providers caring for the transgender population.[15] Most notably, 1 year of hormonal therapy and living as the desired gender is required before gender-confirming (permanent) surgeries. For transgender women (male to female), hormonal therapy includes estrogen supplementation with or without antiandrogen therapy such as spironolactone or cyproterone acetate.[15] The goal of hormonal therapy is to feminize patients by changing fat distribution, decreasing muscle mass, inducing breast formation, reducing testicular size, and reducing male pattern hair growth.[15,16] The rate at which the physical effects occur after estrogen initiation varies, with changes starting within a few months and progressing for 2 to 3 years.[16] Although the physical changes may be striking, they may be too subtle for some patients (**Fig. 1**). Noninvasive aesthetic treatments can further enhance appearance by softening, contouring, and balancing features according to specific aesthetic goals (**Figs. 2–4**).

Transgender men (female to male) may choose to undergo hormonal therapy with exogenous testosterone.[15] Testosterone therapy suppresses

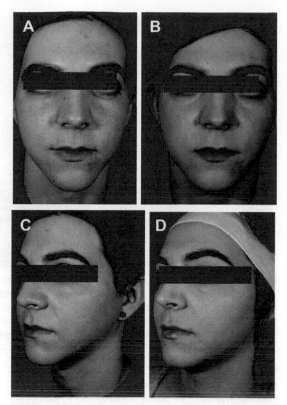

Fig. 1. Before (*A*) and after (*B*) hormonal therapy. Aesthetic changes include wider and more rounded convexities at temple and cheek. Also note the midface appears fuller with a softer and less angular contour through the mandible and chin. Before (*C*) and after (*D*) facial fillers in the same patient reveal more widening at the temple, cheek, and tear trough with a softer and more rounded contour to the mandible chin. The lips are subtly enhanced to reveal a more natural feminine projection with elevated mouth corners.

female secondary sex characteristics and masculinizes transgender men. The effects of testosterone can be seen within 3 months of initiating therapy, including cessation of menses, changes in fat distribution, increases in muscle mass, and increased libido. Changes that occur later include deepened voice, vaginal skin atrophy, and increased clitoral size.[15] Skin effects that occur during this period may include increased facial and body hair, increased acne, and male pattern hair loss.[15]

Surgical procedures are available for transgender patients in addition to medical therapy or if the effects of sex hormone treatment are unsatisfactory.[16] For transgender women, surgical options include genital affirmation surgery to remove the testes (orchiectomy), vaginoplasty (to create a neovagina), breast augmentation surgery,

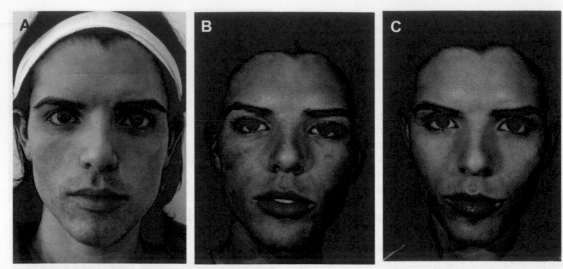

Fig. 2. (A) Before and (B) after laser hair removal to the lower face, showing reduction in shadowing and softening of skin texture. This patient also received injectables to the upper face (A) before and after botulinum toxin to smooth and gently arch the brow and (B) immediately after facial fillers to the midface and lower face to enhance convexity of cheek and lips, and smooth contour of the mandible and chin. (C) After botulinum to the masseter muscle the face appears more heart shaped.

chondrolaryngoplasty for prominent larynx (tracheal shave for Adam's apple), voice feminization surgery, or facial feminization surgeries including rhinoplasty and forehead and chin implants.[16] For transgender men, surgical options include chest masculinization surgery, metoidioplasty, phalloplasty, scrotoplasty, hysterectomy, and oophorectomy.[17]

One recent population study based in Boston Medical Center between 2004 and 1015, published in July 2017, reported that 35% of subjects had undergone at least 1 gender-affirming surgery.[18] Thus, most transgender clinic patients had not undergone any type of gender-affirmation surgery. The low rate may be caused by financial cost, lack of interest, lack of availability, aversion to invasive procedures,[18] or any of the aforementioned barriers to care.

Quality-of-Life Data for Gender Identity and Aesthetic Procedures

Transgender women and men report a lower QOL compared with the general population.[19–21] Both medical hormonal therapy[19] and gender-reaffirming surgeries[20] have been shown to be associated with high satisfaction and higher quality of life. However, even after transitioning, the population remains at risk for lower QOL and mental health.[21] Adjunct minimally invasive aesthetic procedures may assist in the transition process and further increase body image, satisfaction with appearance, and QOL. This

option could be most important for the patients in the first year on hormonal therapy, to ease their gender dysphoria and help them feel more comfortable in their chosen gender identity while they are awaiting gender confirmation surgery.

A recent cross-sectional survey study of 327 people showed that most transgender women thought that their faces were the most essential body part to have changed. Of facial procedures, transgender women reported hair removal was the most important aesthetic procedure, followed by surgery and then injectables.[3] The women reported seeking procedures mostly from plastic surgeons,[3] which may indicate preference, prior therapeutic relationship, marketing/community outreach, or ease of access. In contrast, transgender men were most concerned with their chests, more than their faces or genitals. Patients also reported that their priority with aesthetic procedures is that it looks good, being more important than the risk of scars, complications, or other risks. The authors postulate that minimally invasive aesthetic procedures performed by dermatologists could be more popular in both transgender men and women with more community outreach and literature detailing the available procedures and typical outcomes, thus enhancing safety and reducing the risk of complications in this population. Patients also need before and after images they can relate to, rather than attempting to extrapolate typical results from cisgender patient images.

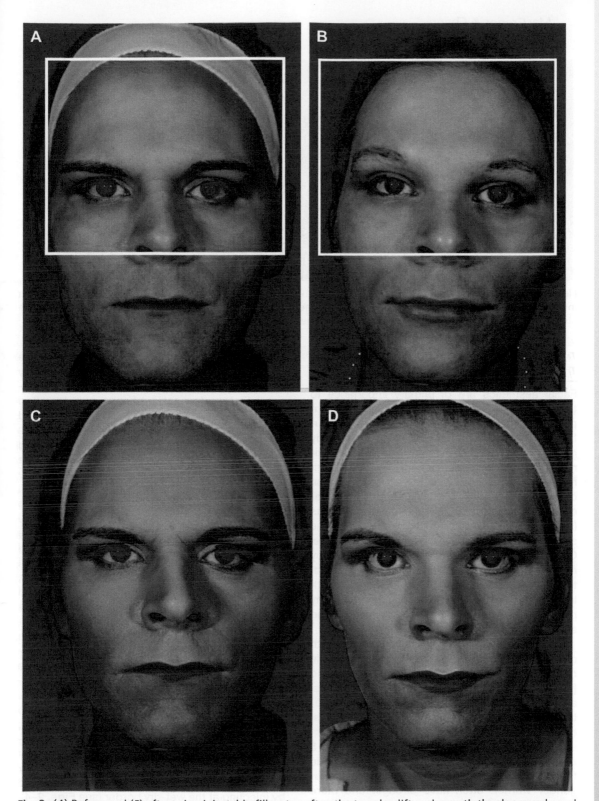

Fig. 3. (*A*) Before and (*B*) after using injectable fillers to soften the temples, lift and smooth the depressed nasal root, and reduce the prominent supraorbital brow ridges (with makeup removed). Additional lift to the brow was achieved after polydioxanone thread lifting, 2 treatments of microfocused ultrasound skin tightening, as well as botulinum toxin injection. (*C*) Before and (*D*) after with makeup showing the overall impact of upper face treatment as well as lower face. The lower face was treated with botulinum toxin injection to masseters to produce a more heart-shaped, tapered jawline and fillers were used to enhance lip volume as well as lift the mouth corners and soften the chin/prejowl sulcus. Note that the lips will be treated in several sessions over time to gradually build volume while preserving a natural shape.

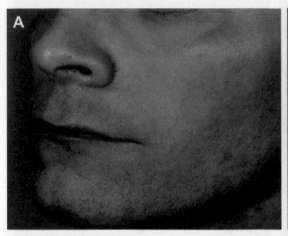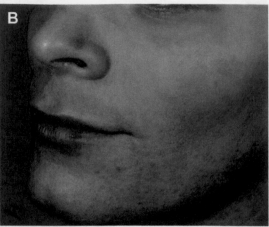

Fig. 4. (*A*) Before and (*B*) after oblique side angle showing the effect of lower face smoothing achieved with injectable facial filler, botulinum toxin, polydioxanone thread lifting, and laser hair removal. The lower face also looks more narrow and lifted in proportion to the upper face.

Transgender Women (Male to Female Transition)

Facial aesthetics are of primary importance to transgender women.[3] The face is the first feature presented to the world and is less easily camouflaged than the chest or genitals. Estrogen therapy may reduce facial hair, but rarely eradicates terminal hairs in the beard distribution, making laser hair removal the first concern for most.[3] Hair reduction on the face smooths the skin and has a major, life-changing impact on appearance in these patients (see **Figs. 2–4**) but often takes more than the average 6 to 8 sessions in the authors' experience. Other changes expected from estrogen therapy may be softening and rounding of the forehead, temple, cheek/midface, and mandible, with less angular features (see **Fig. 1**); however, many patients wish for additional or more rapid enhancements.

Modest facial contouring can be achieved with minimally invasive treatments, such as injectable botulinum toxin, soft tissue fillers, thread lifting (with polydioxanone or poly-L-lactic acid sutures) and energy-based tightening devices. Some patients with prominent supraorbital brow ridges, depressed nasal root, or flat brow benefit from upper face injectable fillers (see **Fig. 4**; **Figs. 5** and **6**), botulinum toxin, thread lifting, and skin tightening in combination. Specifically, transgender women often have stronger and more prominent facial muscles, including the glabellar complex, frontalis, and masseter muscles. These muscles can be treated with botulinum toxin injections to relax and soften them. In the authors' experience, transgender women tend to require a higher dosage than most cisgender women to achieve an adequate response. Long-term use of botulinum toxin also works to chemically shrink these muscles, without the need for surgery. Flat or low-set eyebrows can be lifted and arched by the use of strategically placed botulinum toxin in the glabella, filler injections around and under the brow, thread lifts placed in the forehead from the frontotemporal hairline to lift up, and microfocused ultrasound of the forehead to create a brow lift. Patients with particularly heavy brows or prominent supraorbital brow ridges may elect surgical reduction for more dramatic improvements. For those who transition postpuberty, a flat midface and cheek as well as hollow tear troughs may benefit from lifting and widening to enhance softer, rounder convexities and a more heart-shaped face (see **Figs. 2** and **6**). This outcome can be obtained by filler injections in the cheeks, temples, tear troughs, and forehead to enhance bone structure as well as botulinum toxin injections in the masseters to slim or taper the jawline, thereby creating a heart-shaped, traditionally feminine facial contour (see **Figs. 2–4**). Patients of all gender identities may wish to maintain a stronger or more angular jawline, and this preference should be asked of the patient. Lips can be shaped according to patient preference by manipulating the vermillion border (see **Fig. 1**A, C), and/or enhanced and volumized by injecting at the wet-dry border (see **Figs. 2–4**). The perioral and prejowl area can also be addressed with filler to blend volume and soften harsh angles and shadows as well as to soften the chin (see **Figs. 1–4**). Botulinum toxin injections to the chin can also be used to relax mentalis dimpling.

255

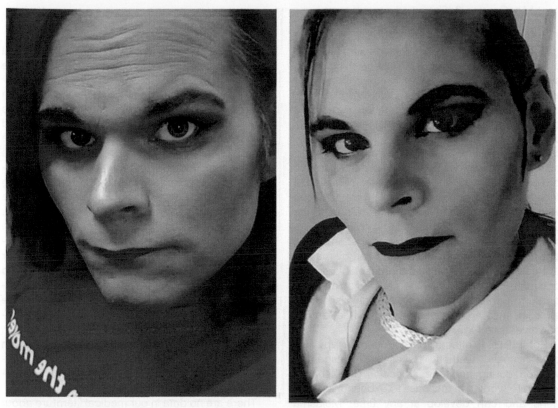

Fig. 5. The patient's own photographs showing the before and after change achieved through minimally invasive aesthetic procedures including injectable fillers, botulinum toxin, microfused ultrasound skin tightening, polydioxanone thread lifting, and laser hair removal.

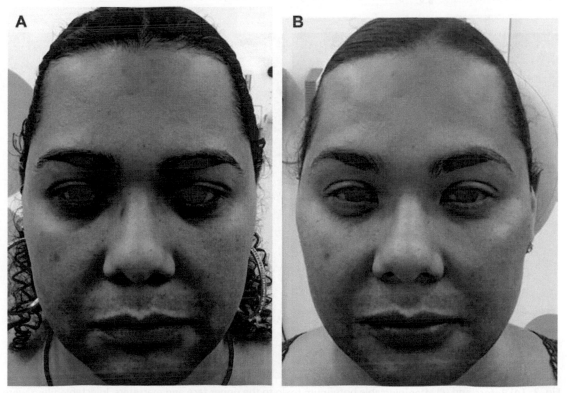

Fig. 6. (*A*) Before and (*B*) after a single session of treatment with little to no downtime. This patient received botulinum toxin to the glabella and injectable filler to lift the tear trough and enhance convexities of the cheek and temple.

Some transgender women present already pleased with their features, just wishing for a smaller correction to enhance their beauty or emphasize certain features. Cultural influences, personal preferences, or simply any person's own unique aesthetic can influence the desired outcome. **Fig. 7** shows how small tweaks or details can enhance beauty and improve proportions. This patient wished for a more taut, arched brow and a more tapered jawline, revealing a more heart-shaped face; her goals were achieved with a single session of injectable botulinum to the upper face and masseters along with facial fillers to the temples, cheeks, mouth corners, and body of the lip. Improving facial proportions by making the upper face wider, lifting the nasolabial angle, or small volume filler to the nasal root or nasal dorsum (nonsurgical rhinoplasty) can also make a larger nose appear smaller, more lifted, and/or narrower (see **Figs. 4, 5**, and **7**)

Potential side effects from estrogen therapy also present new aesthetic issues for transgender women during and after transition. Melasma is known to worsen in response to exogenous estrogens and can develop at any time. Melasma partially responds to maintenance topical therapy with daily application of mineral sunscreens, retinoids, hydroquinone, botanic brighteners, antioxidants, and peeling agents. Low-density,

low-energy 1927-nm fractional resurfacing several times per year is also an option to accelerate brightening of pigmentation and maintain remission. New leg veins secondary to estrogen can be treated with sclerotherapy and lasers, whereas new-onset cellulite can be temporarily smoothed with radiofrequency-based energy devices. Striae can be treated with vascular lasers, nonablative fractional resurfacing, microneedling, or combination. Estrogen therapy does not alter a receding hairline. Topical minoxidil and platelet-rich plasma are treatment options for androgenetic alopecia, which may be continued in transgender women to prevent worsening of hairline recession. Transgender women may want to consider follicular unit hair transplant to restore a lower hairline and to cover a thinning vertex, especially if longer hairstyles are desired. In some of our patients, we have also seen a loss of mandibular size and structure following estrogen therapy. The resulting skin laxity and submental adiposity may benefit from skin tightening with radiofrequency or microfocused ultrasound and fat reduction with cryolipolysis or deoxycholate injections, respectively.

There are no data in our medical literature about transgender women's body contouring attitudes and preferences. In the authors' experience, the abdomen, flanks, inner thighs, and bra line adiposity all respond well to cryolipolysis, pulsed

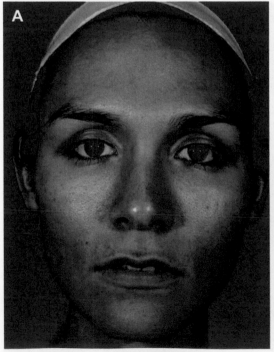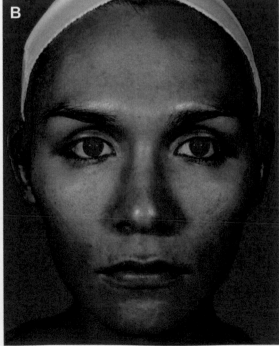

Fig. 7. (*A*) Before and (*B*) after injectable botulinum toxin to the upper face and masseters. Injectable fillers were placed to widen the temples and cheeks as well as lift the mouth corners and plump the body of the lip.

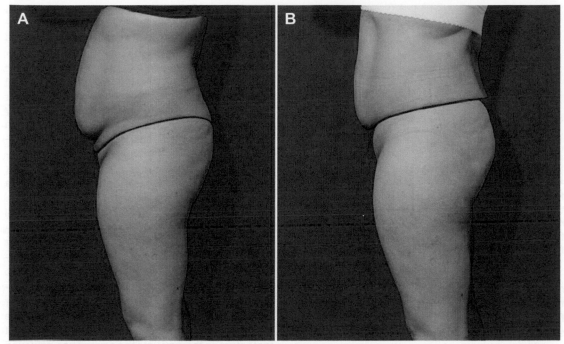

Fig. 8. (*A*) Before and (*B*) 2 months after abdominal Cryolipolysis combined with 3 twice-monthly sessions of pulsed forced ultrasonography in transgender woman.

focused ultrasound, and/or radiofrequency body contouring devices (**Fig. 8**). Hip and buttock augmentation may be desired and could be obtained through filler injections, but the volume of product required over several sessions proves to be cost-prohibitive for most (making this procedure rare in our office).[9,11] For the hip and buttock, fat harvesting and transplant could be another option. Breast augmentation through surgical correction (top surgery) and vaginoplasty (bottom surgery) yields some degree of scarring in most

patients. If the scars are undesirable, vascular laser, resurfacing, or microneedling with radiofrequency can be considered (**Figs. 9** and **10**).

Transgender Men (Female to Male Transition)

Although transgender men are more concerned with their chests than their faces or genitals, dermatologic care and noninvasive treatments are of benefit in these patients. In the authors' experience, pseudogynecomastia (residual breast tissue) still present after testosterone therapy does

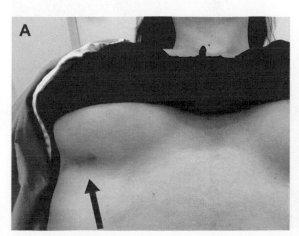
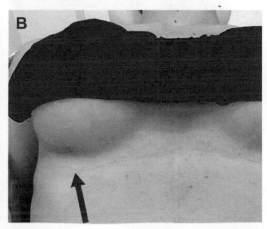

Fig. 9. (*A*) Before and (*B*) after 2 sessions of nonablative fractional laser resurfacing to blend breast augmentation scars in a transgender woman.

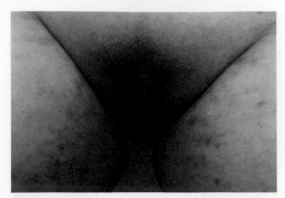

Fig. 10. Postoperative result of vaginoplasty in a transgender woman. Scars are not noticeable and require no treatment. She was recently treated for folliculitis and will first receive a topical regimen to fade resulting pigmentation.

not respond well to minimally invasive aesthetic treatment, and we routinely refer these patients for surgical correction (**Fig. 11**). On the face, some transgender men wish to maintain new hair growth or shave, whereas others in our care have sought laser hair removal of new facial hair experienced after testosterone therapy. Noninvasive body contouring, particularly on the abdomen, flanks, and submental adiposity, should also be considered in transgender men.

Although possibly not the top concern, many transgender men also present for enhancements to facial contour. We have seen many transgender men who benefit from facial injectables to refine facial features. On the upper face, botulinum can be used to flatten and strengthen the brow, whereas injectable fillers can be used on the mid-face and lower face to refine a more prominent and angular zygoma, mandible, and chin (**Fig. 12**). Some patients also note that bone structure fluctuates slightly during cyclic testosterone injection cycles, and we recommend photographs, examination, and treatment follow-up at several weekly time points to achieve the desired end point with facial contouring in transgender men. As previously discussed, testosterone-related acne, folliculitis, pigmentation, and scarring can be severe. Dermatologists are the experts and can play a supportive role by managing acne and folliculitis. Scarring and pigmentation can be reduced in all skin types by topical retinoids, peeling, and brightening agents, as well as multiple fractional laser resurfacing and microneedling with radiofrequency treatments in series. In patients who note accelerated male-patterned, or androgenetic, alopecia during and after transition, follicular unit hair transplant should be considered. Finasteride should not be considered in the first 2 years of testosterone therapy until the patient has achieved their desired secondary sex characteristics.

Nonbinary Gender Status

There is increased awareness about individuals who do not identify specifically with either gender (nonbinary or intersex) thanks to educational media campaigns,[22,23] attention in art/film,[24] and public political struggles.[25] This nonbinary status could be related to intersex or ambiguous genitalia at birth, personal preference, or both. Many

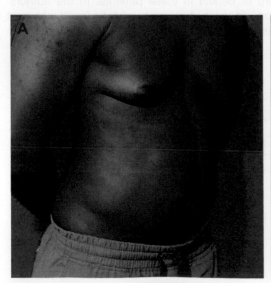
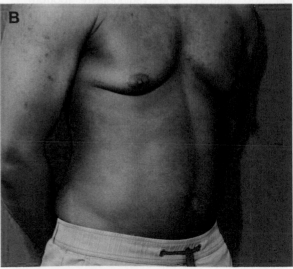

Fig. 11. Transgender man (A) before and (B) after Cryolipolysis to the chest. No change is seen and the patient ultimately sought surgical correction.

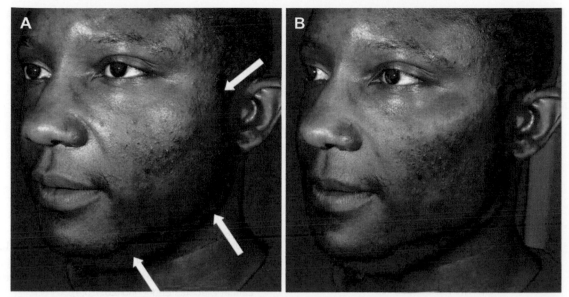

Fig. 12. (A) Before (arrows indicate areas where structure was enhanced with injectable filler) and (B) immediately after a single session of facial fillers to strengthen and contour the temple, zygoma, mandible, and chin with calcium hydroxylapatite. Testosterone-induced acne is also seen and the patient has started topical retinoids and a brightening/peeling regimen.

advocates think that people in this category should not have surgical intervention in infancy or childhood[24,25] and should be allowed to choose their gender identities themselves after puberty in early adulthood or remain intersex over the long term. In medical offices, all electronic and paper forms should be inclusive and easy to navigate for all gender identities. Patients should be asked which pronouns they prefer and told to fill out forms however they wish or however they identify. Providers should never assume that any individual wishes to receive traditionally masculinizing or feminizing procedures. As with any patient, physicians should ask open-ended questions while viewing their mirror reflection (eg, "Tell me you see," or "What would you like to achieve," or even "What do you love and want to accentuate") and listen carefully to each patient's aesthetic aspirations. It is also important to remember that viewing their own clinical photographs may be psychologically difficult at times (always ask first whether they want to see their images before showing them). Treatment recommendations are then guided by the practitioner's suggestions and continually modified as the patient provides feedback.

SUMMARY

As the number of people seeking gender transition grows, the importance of dermatologists in facilitating this transition process in a safe and smooth manner also increases. Dermatologists may offer much speedier access to minimally invasive procedures that make a significant difference in the confidence and QOL of transgender patients. To that effect, more dermatologic literature is needed on the best, safest treatments that can be provided to patients. Clinicians must also coordinate with transgender patients, medical endocrinologists, and surgeons during the transition process. Staff should be well trained and office procedures should be modified to be inclusive of transgender men, women, and nonbinary gender status individuals. Rather than being all-assuming, the authors recommend being open with patients about their preferred use of pronouns, names, as well as their aesthetic preferences. It is important to understand that everyone experiences transitioning differently, and rather than clinging to paternalistic tendencies, physicians need to listen and accommodate the needs of their patients. Open-minded listening and regularly asking for preferences help cultivate a respectful relationship. To that point, when we ask our transgender patients, "What do you wish doctors would do differently when you seek their help?" we hear repeatedly, "I feel that doctors should listen more than talk and try to understand where the patient is coming from rather than their own opinions. Everyone's journey is different." We hope this article is the first of many steps to understanding and providing the best care for transgender and nonbinary patients.

REFERENCES

1. Estimates of transgender populations in states with legislation impacting transgender people (update): how many adults identify as transgender in the United States? In: The Williams Institute UCLA School of Law. 2016. Available at: http://williamsinstitute.law.ucla.edu/wp-content/uploads/How-Many-Adults-Identify-as-Transgender-in-the-United-States.pdf. Accessed November 11 2018.

2. Estimates of transgender populations in states with legislation impacting transgender people (Update): age of individuals who identify as transgender in the United States. In: The Williams Institute UCLA School of Law. 2017. Available at: https://williamsinstitute.law.ucla.edu/wp-content/uploads/TransAgeReport.pdf. Accessed November 11, 2018.

3. Ginsberg BA, Calderon M, Seminara NM, et al. A potential role for the dermatologist in the physical transformation of transgender people: a survey of attitudes and practices within the transgender community. J Am Acad Dermatol 2016;74:303–8.

4. Boos MD, Ginsberg BA, Peebles JK. Prescribing isotretinoin to transgender youth: a pledge for more inclusive care. Pediatr Dermatol 2019;36(1):169–71.

5. Wierckx K, Van de Peer F, Verhaeghe E, et al. Short- and long-term clinical skin effects of testosterone treatment in trans men. J Sex Med 2014;11(1):222–9.

6. Carruthers JD, Glogau RG, Blitzer A. Facial aesthetics consensus group faculty. Advances in facial rejuvenation: botulinum type a, hyaluronic acid dermal fillers and combination therapies-consensus recommendations. Plast Reconstr Surg 2008;121(5Suppl):5S–30S.

7. Altman K. Facial feminization surgery: current state of the art. Int J Oral Maxillofac Surg 2012;41(8):885–94.

8. Ascha M, Swanson MA, Massie JP, et al. Nonsurgical management of facial masculinization and feminization. Aesthet Surg J 2019;39(5):123–37.

9. Walker H. Body of work: from DIY hormones to silicone injections, why some trans women choose to transition outside the medical industry. Out magazine 2019;75–8.

10. Murariu D, Holland MC, Gampper TJ, et al. Illegal silicone injections create unique reconstructive challenges in transgender patients. Plast Reconstr Surg 2015;135(5):932e–3e.

11. Pinto TP, Teixeira FDB, Barros CRDS, et al. Use of industrial liquid silicone to transform the body: prevalence and factors associated with its use among transvestites and transsexual women in São Paulo, Brazil. Cad Saude Publica 2017;33(7):1–13.

12. Sobanko JF, Dai J, Gelfand JM, et al. Prospective cohort study investigating changes in body image, quality of life and self esteem following minimally invasive cosmetic procedures. Dermatol Surg 2018;44(8):1121–8.

13. Marks DH, Awosika O, Rengifo-Pardo M, et al. Dermatologic surgical care for transgender individuals. Dermatol Surg 2019;45(3):446–57.

14. White Hughto JM, Reisner SL, Pachankis JE. Transgender stigma and health: a critical review of stigma determinants, mechanisms, and interventions. Soc Sci Med 2015;147:222–31.

15. Unger CA. Hormone therapy for transgender patients. Transl Androl Urol 2016;5(6):877–84.

16. Tangpricha V, den Heijer M. Oestrogen and anti-androgen therapy for transgender women. Lancet Diabetes Endocrinol 2017;5(4):291–300.

17. Irwig MS. Testosterone therapy for transgender men. Lancet Diabetes Endocrinol 2017;5(4):301–11.

18. Kailas M, Lu HMS, Rothman EF, et al. Prevalence and types of gender-affirming surgery among a sample of transgender endocrinology patients prior to state expansion of insurance coverage. Endocr Pract 2017;23(7):780–6.

19. Gorin-Lazard A, Baumstarck K, Boyer L, et al. Is hormonal therapy associated with better quality of life in transsexuals? A cross-sectional study. J Sex Med 2012;9(2):531–41.

20. Wierckx K, Van Caenegem E, Elaut E, et al. Quality of life and sexual health after sex reassignment surgery in transsexual men. J Sex Med 2011;8(12):3379–88.

21. Jellestad L, Jäggi T, Corbisiero S, et al. Quality of life in transitioned trans persons: a retrospective cross-sectional cohort study. Biomed Res Int 2018;2018:8684625.

22. These activists get real about being intersex. In: Teen Vogue June 2017. Available at: https://video.teenvogue.com/watch/these-activists-get-real-about-being-intersex. Accessed on April 10, 2019.

23. Common misconceptions about sex and gender. In: Teen Vogue March 2019. Available at: https://video.teenvogue.com/watch/5-common-misconceptions-about-sex-and-gender. Accessed on April 10, 2019.

24. About river Gallo and Ponyboi the film. Available at: https://www.rivergallo.com/about. Accessed on April 10, 2019.

25. California becomes the first state to condemn intersex surgeries on children. In: USA Today August 28, 2018. Available at: https://www.usatoday.com/story/news/nation/2018/08/28/intersex-surgeries-children-california-first-state-condemn/1126185002/. Accessed on April 10, 2019.

Surgical Facial Esthetics for Gender Affirmation

Jonathan M. Sykes, MD[a,b],*, Amanda E. Dilger, MD[c], Alexander Sinclair, MD[d,1]

KEYWORDS

• Facial feminization • Transgender surgery • Facial plastic surgery • Rhinoplasty • Facial anatomy

KEY POINTS

- The appearance and beauty of the face is a complex combination of the size, shape, and orientation of multiple layers of the face, including the bone, muscle, fat, and skin.
- The sexual identity of an individual is easily very obvious to most observers with only a quick glance or when only noticing a small portion of the face. Even though the overall appearance of the male face is quite different (and easily noticeable) from the female face, the differences in different facial structures—such as the brow bone, chin, nose, or lips—can be quite small.
- It is the sum of all of these small, yet measurable differences, that creates the obvious dimorphism in facial appearance.

INTRODUCTION

The appearance and beauty of the face is a complex combination of the size, shape, and orientation of multiple layers of the face, including the bone, muscle, fat, and skin. The overall facial structure of an individual is a composite of genetics, embryology, and heredity.

The sexual identity of an individual is very obvious to most observers with only a quick glance or when only noticing a small portion of the face. Even though the overall appearance of the male face is quite different (and easily noticeable) from the female face, the differences in different facial structures—such as the brow bone, chin, nose, or lips—can be quite small. It is the sum of all of these small, yet measurable differences, that creates the obvious dimorphism in facial appearance.

This article outlines the anthropometric sexual differences between facial features and discusses surgical procedures designed to alter the facial appearance and facial sexual identity. The individual patient needs, the diagnosis of facial dimorphism, and the limitations of these techniques are outlined.

SEXUAL DIFFERENCES IN FACIAL APPEARANCE

The recognition of an individual's sexual identity based on facial appearance occurs at a subconscious level and relies on several physical features that are characteristically gender specific. Facial recognition studies in psychology literature have demonstrated that although individuals are consistently able to identify a subject as a man or woman based on eyes or lips alone, masking of the eyes, lips or nose of the subject causes a significant delay in timing of sex recognition. The effect of masking on delayed or loss of ability to identify sex was postulated not to be due to the loss of the individual feature per se, but because of the disruption in the relationship between the structure and the remaining facial anatomy.[1,2]

[a] Facial Plastic Surgery, UC Davis Medical Center, Sacramento, CA, USA; [b] Facial Plastic Surgery, Roxbury Institute, Beverly Hills, CA, USA; [c] Facial Plastic and Reconstructive Surgery, 5 Medical Plaza, Suite 100. Roseville, CA 95661, USA; [d] Transgender Center, Southern California Hospital System, Culver City, CA, USA
[1] Present address: 9001 Wilshire Boulevard, Suite 202, Beverly Hills, CA 90211.
* Corresponding author. 5 Medical Plaza, Suite 100, Roseville, CA 95661.
E-mail address: jmsykes@ucdavis.edu

Dermatol Clin 38 (2020) 261–268
https://doi.org/10.1016/j.det.2019.10.011
0733-8635/20/© 2019 Elsevier Inc. All rights reserved.

The variations in anatomy of male and female faces are seen at every level—from skin and soft tissue to fat density and volume to muscles and bone structure. As a result, there are anatomic sexual dimorphisms in the upper, middle, and lower third of the face as well as the neck that are of variable in prominence in different individuals. Management of facial esthetics in the transgender patient requires a thorough understanding of the anatomy underlying these gender-specific characteristics. Once the anatomy is understood, an individualized approach to gender-affirming facial surgery can be developed that is suitable to each patient's existing anatomy and goals for transformation.

HAIRLINE, FOREHEAD, AND BROWS

A masculine versus feminine appearance of the upper third of the face is affected by the position and shape of the hairline and by the contour and height of the forehead. Female hairlines are typically situated lower than the hairline of males. Although forehead height is variable in all individuals, female forehead height is approximately 5.5 to 5.8 cm above the eyebrows. On the other hand, the male forehead height averages 7 to 8 cm above the brows. Of course, some men exhibit androgenic alopecia with aging, which can result in temporal recession and loss of hair in the frontal hairline. In these individuals, the height of the forehead lengthens with aging.

The other difference that exists in the men versus women is hairline shape. The male hairline is more likely to show temporal hairline recession. The central hairline also exhibits some sexual dimorphism. A widow's peak is present in approximately 81% of female hairlines.[3,4] This makes the central forehead lower in women who have this trait.

The largest difference in forehead appearance is in overall shape. The bony contour of the male forehead is more convex than is the forehead in women. The forehead in women is, therefore, generally shorter as well as flatter, whereas male foreheads tend to have a convexity at the supraorbital rim. These dimorphisms can be addressed in the male patient transitioning to female with hairline lowering, forehead height shortening, and bony contouring of the prominent forehead and supraorbital rim.

Hairline-lowering procedures will not only advance the frontal hairline, but will also shorten the forehead height. This will affect the perceived size of the face. It is important to take into account the patient's relative midface size and height. Scalp laxity must also be assessed. Scalps that are relatively immobile require significant advancement, which usually requires multiple galeotomies. If scalp mobility is inadequate, the amount of hairline advancement may be limited. Patients with significant temporal recession may also benefit from hair transplantation, which may be performed at the time of the forehead and brow surgery, or may be delayed for several months.

Masculine foreheads can exhibit significant frontal bossing, which is a result of either a large frontal sinus or thickened supraorbital rim. Therefore, the nasofrontal angle tends to be more acute in men and more obtuse in women.[5–7] This trait may give the sense of deeper set eyes in men.

SURGICAL FOREHEAD FEMINIZATION

There are 4 variations of forehead feminization procedures. These subtypes were initially described by Ousterhout in 1987[8] and are contingent on a patient's individual forehead anatomy. For all surgical forehead feminization procedures, access is achieved via a coronal or trichophytic incision. The decision on which type of incision to make is based on whether the patient is undergoing a concurrent hairline lowering procedure. If hairline lowering is indicated, a trichophytic incision is made following the temporal hairline as described above. The scalp is injected with standard tumescent solution and dissection is carried out in the subperiosteal plane to the level of the frontal processes of the zygomas bilaterally, exposing the entire supraorbital rim and extending 1 cm onto the roof of the orbit. The supraorbital nerve is dissected to fully expose the supraorbital rim.[5]

A type I forehead consists of a forehead that does not have a frontal sinus or had a sufficiently thick frontal sinus. This is rare and is described in only 3% to 5% of patients undergoing facial feminization procedures.[4,8] In these patients, frontal bossing can be addressed with burring and without osteotomies.[9]

With the type II forehead, the glabella is in good anterior-posterior position and can be shaped with burring without osteotomies; however, the depression cephalad to the glabella requires augmentation. This is extensively described by Ousterhout using methyl methacrylate implants[10] and in more recent literature with soft expanded polytetrafluoroethylene and silicone implants.[11] Injectable fillers are another option for forehead augmentation; however, the injector must be careful to avoid the supratrochlear and supraorbital neurovascular bundles given the rare but serious risk of necrosis or blindness. The needle should be introduced lateral to the supraorbital foramen (1 fingerbreadth lateral from the medial canthus, mean 10.8 ± 4.9 mm) and advanced gently deep to the frontalis and superficial to the periosteum. Injection should be made in a slow retrograde technique starting medial to the medial canthus to avoid the deep branch of the supratrochlear artery.[12]

The type III forehead is the most common, occurring in 93% of patients in 1 study,[4] and technically the most challenging as it requires removal and reshaping of the anterior table of the frontal sinus. Computerized tomography (CT) scanning of the sinuses should be used preoperatively to plan the location of the osteotomies (**Fig. 1**) and assess any asymmetry in the sinuses. When removing the anterior table, it is important to preserve the remaining mucosa of the frontal sinus. After shaping the anterior table, it is replaced and secured using 3 titanium miniplates (**Fig. 2**). These patients typically also require contouring of the outer third of the superior orbital rim with a burr.

A type IV forehead is rarely encountered and is described as a small forehead with an underprojected brow that requires augmentation. The techniques used for augmentation are similar to those described for the type II forehead and are applied in the supraorbital and glabellar region as well as in the adjacent cephalad forehead.

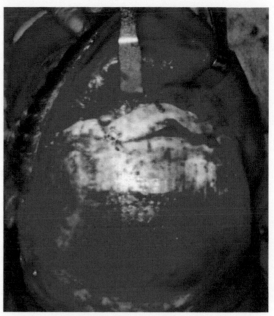

Fig. 2. The reshaped portion of the anterior table is replaced and secured with 3 titanium miniplates.

Eyebrow position and shape can contribute significantly to the determination of gender by facial characteristics.[13] Although hair on the eyebrow can be greatly affected by stylization, trimming, and application of make-up, female brows are typically higher and more arched than brows of male patients. Female brows are typically slightly above the supraorbital rim, whereas male brows are positioned on the supraorbital rim. Therefore, a brow lift is often performed in conjunction with hairline lowering, orbital rim contouring, and forehead feminization procedures to feminize the brow position.

THE NOSE AND MIDFACE

As discussed previously, men typically have a more acute nasofrontal angle than women. This is in part caused by characteristic frontal bossing in men. Frontal bossing can be treated with forehead and supraorbital rim contouring procedures. If the frontonasal transition also needs to be lowered, this can be accomplished using a rounded or conical burr. This will then determine the height of the nasal dorsum for the rhinoplasty.

In general, the female nose is smaller than the male nose and is characterized by a straight or concave profile with a vertically and horizontally lower nasion, increased rotation, and a more refined nasal tip.[14] Feminization of the nose thus usually involves standard reduction rhinoplasty

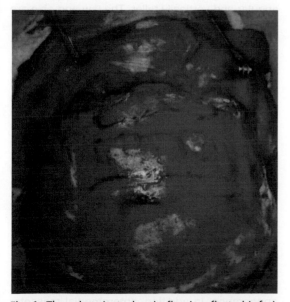

Fig. 1. The subperiosteal scalp flap is reflected inferiorly to expose the anterior table of the frontal bone and supraorbital rim. Osteotomy sites are marked based on preoperative evaluation with a CT scan.

techniques, which can be performed through either an endonasal or open approach.

Tip refinement is an important component in feminization rhinoplasty. To achieve an esthetically appealing tip with long-term stability, the surgeon must balance cartilage removal with grafts and suturing. When removing a cephalic strip of the lower lateral cartilages, for example, it is important to leave at least 6 mm of lateral crura to avoid collapse. Intradomal and interdomal sutures between the medial and lateral crura will help achieve optimal tip rotation, projection, and refinement, as well as stabilize the new nasal tip. Grafts, such as columellar struts and caudal extension grafts can be added in a tongue-in-groove fashion to the septal cartilage.

Reduction of a dorsal hump or a high dorsum to feminize the profile is achieved by removal of bone or cartilage. For a hump that is larger than 2 mm, a Rubin or Cinelli osteotome is used. It is crucial that the osteotome is angled toward the glabella to avoid overresection and creation of a step-off in the dorsum. For smaller humps or dorsal irregularities, a Fomon rasp may be used. If a significant amount of bone or cartilage has been removed, it is important to address the resultant open roof deformity. This can be done in a variety of ways, including with spreader grafts between the upper lateral cartilages and septum, spreader flaps, and reapproximation of the upper lateral cartilages.[15]

Augmentation of the cheeks with implants or injectable filler contributes to a feminine appearance by triangulating the lower two-thirds of the face with the base of the triangle at the lateral aspects of the cheek and the apex at the chin point. High-density polyethylene implants are available in several different shapes and sizes and can be placed easily through an intraoral incision. An appropriately sized pocket is dissected along the zygomatic arches and, once optimal symmetry is confirmed, the implants are secured to the zygoma with 2-mm titanium screws of at least 6 mm in length.[5]

LIPS

In women, the upper lip is generally shorter and fuller with an accentuated philtral dimple and defined, everted vermillion border. Therefore, there may be more maxillary display of teeth in women than in men.[5] Feminization of the lip therefore typically involves reduction of lip height with augmentation to increase lip fullness and visibility of the vermillion border.[4] This is achieved surgically through a lip-lift via the modified bullhorn technique. Local anesthesia is injected in the standard fashion, then a premeasured ellipse of skin and subcutaneous tissue is excised immediately adjacent to the sill between the alar bases. In general, no more than 25% of the height from the nasal sill to the vermillion border is excised. A variety of techniques for lip augmentation have been described, including dermis grafting to plump the vermillion border,[5] hyaluronic acid lip filler, and autologous fat transfer.[16]

If both a lip-lift and an open rhinoplasty (with significant dissection of the columella) are to be performed, these 2 procedures should be staged to avoid necrosis in the segment of skin between the traditional columellar incision and the lip-lift incision. The lip-lift can be safely performed at the same time with an endonasal rhinoplasty.

MANDIBLE AND JAWLINE

The male mandible is generally wider with a more prominent angle (gonial angle). In addition, there is often lipping of the bone in men secondary to attachments of the masseter muscle. The chin in men tends to be more angular and elongated than the female chin. The female chin is usually shorter and more pointed than the chin of males.[17] As a result, the overall female face shape is generally more of a heart or inverted triangle, with the pogonion representing the apex of the triangle. The male face shape is more rectangular and vertically taller. The jaw and chin are usually treated simultaneously such that the changes in jaw contour and chin proportions are complementary.

The masculine jawline is addressed during facial feminization surgery, with the mandible angle being surgically reduced and tapered. An intraoral incision is made to widely expose the angle and body of the mandible, taking care to strip off the pterygomasseteric attachments to the lower border of the jaw. This maneuver helps to minimize bleeding from inadvertent muscle damage during bony contouring. The cortical bone is then reduced, often to the level of cancellous bone, from the prominence of the angle to the mental foramen (**Fig. 3**). It is important to avoid exposure of the tooth roots and the inferior alveolar nerve. In cases where the mandible is significantly angulated, the angle may be osteotomized to achieve a more rounded appearance. In addition, anteromedial masseter muscle resection[5] or masseteric botulinum toxin injection can be used to further soften the appearance of the jawline.[16]

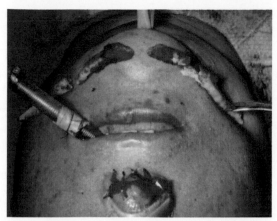

Fig. 3. Patient status after jawline feminization with the osteotomized mandibular bone held adjacent to the new jawline, which has been narrowed and softened.

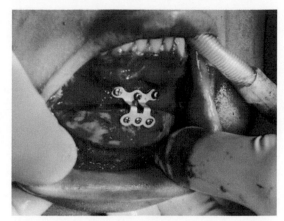

Fig. 4. Titanium miniplate placement after osseous genioplasty.

The goal of the feminization genioplasty is generally to create a smaller and more refined chin. The surgical procedure performed is individualized to the desire of the patient and to their preoperative chin appearance. In most cases, feminization of the chin involves reducing the projection of the chin, narrowing the chin, and shortening of the chin. Osteotomies are generally preferred to bony contouring or implants, because this allows for modification of anterior projection and vertical height simultaneously. An incision is made in the gingivolabial sulcus and dissection is carried out in the subperiosteal plane to expose the chin and inferior border of the mandible, taking care to avoid damage to the mental nerves. Horizontal osteotomies are made with a reciprocating saw. If the vertical height is to be shortened, an ostectomy and wedge of bone is removed. To narrow the chin, a piece of bone is removed from the midline and the 2 lateral fragments are medialized. The chin is then secured in place with titanium miniplates and screws (**Fig. 4**).

THE NECK

In men, the thyroid cartilage is generally larger and more prominent than that of women. The laryngeal prominence (also known as the "Adam's apple," which is formed by the fusion of the 2 thyroid cartilage laminae), is more anteriorly projected in men than in women. This is because the laminae diverge at approximately 90° in men as opposed to approximately 120° in women. Feminization of the thyroid cartilage therefore involves reducing the size of the laryngeal prominence to create a more obtuse angle.

A 2-cm transverse incision is made in the midline neck inferior to the thyroid notch. The perichondrium is incised and dissected to expose the laryngeal prominence and notch. Care must be taken to avoid entering the thyrohyoid membrane. The superior portions of the laminae are then reduced with Rongeurs or a small trimming burr.[5] The result is a less-projected and less-prominent thyroid cartilage.

ADJUNCTIVE ESTHETIC SURGERY

Although some patients present for facial feminization surgery at a younger age, others present later in life and therefore have concomitant aging issues. Patients that have both facial aging as well as gender issues would often benefit from adjunctive esthetic surgery, such as facelift, autologous fat grafting, and/or periorbital and eyelid rejuvenation procedures. There are several benefits to combining feminization and aging procedures including minimizing anesthetic time and cost, maximizing surgical efficiency, and having 1 recovery period. In addition, as patients are generally advised by their endocrinologist to hold hormone replacement therapy for 2 weeks before surgery and 1 week after surgery, combining procedures allows patients to minimize interruptions in their medication regimen. In terms of safety, there has been no demonstrated increased risk of complications related to the vascular supply of the flaps despite elevating multiple planes at once.[18]

Alternatively, there are descriptions in the literature of staging these procedures by facial region (step 1: maxillomandibular complex, nose, and zygoma; step 2: forehead and orbit) and performing the procedures 6 months apart. By achieving a good mandibular dentoskeletal relationship and optimizing the proportions of the inferior and middle third of the face, the groundwork for further esthetic surgery is set by the first step. In addition, staging the facial procedures allows for concomitant genital reassignment surgery, which hastens the overall gender transition process.[19]

CASES AND DISCUSSION

The first case (**Fig. 5**) is of a male-to-female transgender woman who underwent hairline lowering, forehead feminization, brow lift, rhinoplasty, jawline feminization, and genioplasty. The second case (**Fig. 6**) shows a male-to-female transgender woman who underwent hairline lowering, forehead feminization, brow lift, rhinoplasty, lateral mandible shave, and genioplasty. In both cases, an optimal outcome was achieved by addressing the patients' masculine characteristics in the upper, middle, and lower third of the face. The key to surgical planning for these patients is an understanding of the anatomy that underlies the gender-specific features that are to be addressed. With a thorough knowledge of this anatomy, an individualized approach to gender-affirming surgery can be developed to address each patient's goals for transformation.

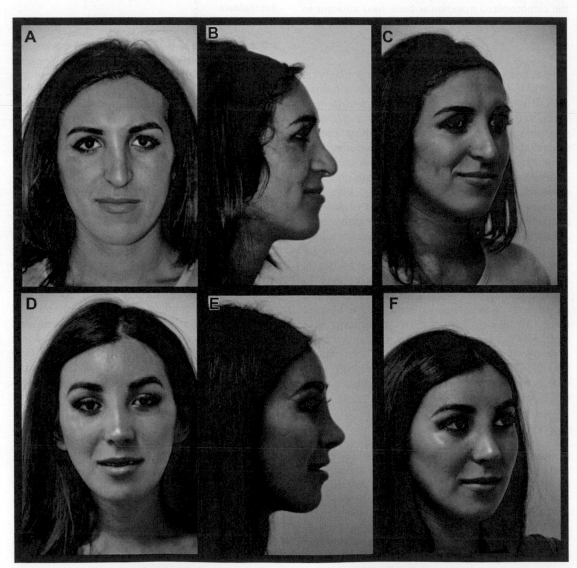

Fig. 5. Frontal, lateral, and oblique preoperative (*A–C*) and postoperative (*D–F*) photographs of a patient (case no. 1) who underwent several facial feminization procedures including hairline advancement, forehead feminization, brow lift, rhinoplasty, cheek implants, mandible angle shaving, and genioplasty.

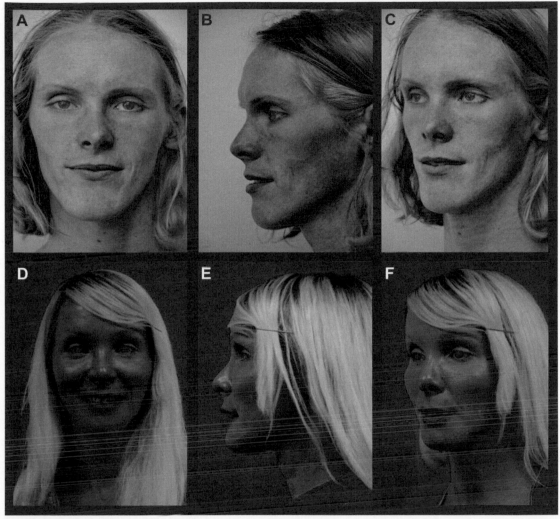

Fig. 6. Frontal, lateral, and oblique preoperative (*A–C*) and postoperative (*D–F*) photographs of a male-to-female transgender patient (case no. 2) who underwent hairline lowering, forehead feminization, brow lift, rhinoplasty, lateral mandible shave, and genioplasty.

DISCLOSURE

The authors have nothing to disclose.

REFERENCES

1. Roberts T, Bruce V. Feature saliency in judging the sex and familiarity of faces. Perception 1988;17(4): 475–81.
2. Bruce V, Burton AM, Hanna E, et al. Sex discrimination: how do we tell the difference between male and female faces? Perception 1993;22(2):131–52.
3. Nusbaum BP, Fuentefria S. Naturally occurring female hairline patterns. Dermatol Surg 2009;35(6): 907–13.
4. Deschamps-Braly JC. Facial gender confirmation surgery: facial feminization surgery and facial

masculinization surgery. Clin Plast Surg 2018; 45(3):323–31.
5. Altman K. Facial feminization surgery: current state of the art. Int J Oral Maxillofac Surg 2012;41(8):885–94.
6. Farkas LG, Kolar JC. Anthropometric guidelines in cranio-orbital surgery. Clin Plast Surg 1987;14(1):1–16.
7. Hwang HS, Kim WS, McNamara JA Jr. Ethnic differences in the soft tissue profile of Korean and European-American adults with normal occlusions and well-balanced faces. Angle Orthod 2002;72(1): 72–80.
8. Ousterhout DK. Feminization of the forehead: contour changing to improve female aesthetics. Plast Reconstr Surg 1987;79(5):701–13.
9. Ousterhout DK. Feminization surgery: a guide for the transgendered woman. Omaha (NE): Addicus Books; 2010.

10. Ousterhout DK, Zlotolow IM. Aesthetic improvement of the forehead utilizing methylmethacrylate onlay implants. Aesthetic Plast Surg 1990;14(4):281–5.

11. Wong JK. Forehead augmentation with alloplastic implants. Facial Plast Surg Clin North Am 2010; 18(1):71–7.

12. Cong LY, Phothong W, Lee SH, et al. Topographic analysis of the supratrochlear artery and the supra-orbital artery: implication for improving the safety of forehead augmentation. Plast Reconstr Surg 2017;139(3):620e–7e.

13. Spiegel JH. Facial determinants of female gender and feminizing forehead cranioplasty. Laryngoscope 2011;121(2):250–61.

14. Springer IN, Zernial O, Nolke F, et al. Gender and nasal shape: measures for rhinoplasty. Plast Reconstr Surg 2008;121(2):629–37.

15. Bellinga RJ, Capitan L, Simon D, et al. Technical and clinical considerations for facial feminization surgery with rhinoplasty and related procedures. JAMA Facial Plast Surg 2017;19(3):175–81.

16. Ascha M, Swanson MA, Massie JP, et al. Nonsurgical management of facial masculinization and feminization. Aesthet Surg J 2019;39(5): NP123–37.

17. Ousterhout D. Feminization of the chin: a review of 485 consecutive cases, vol. 10. Bologna (Italy): Medimond International Proceedings; 2003.

18. Gupta N, Wulu J, Spiegel JH. Safety of combined facial plastic procedures affecting multiple planes in a single setting in facial feminization for transgender patients. Aesthetic Plast Surg 2019;43(4): 993–9.

19. Raffaini M, Magri AS, Agostini T. Full facial feminization surgery: patient satisfaction assessment based on 180 procedures involving 33 consecutive patients. Plast Reconstr Surg 2016;137(2): 438–48.

Ways to Improve Care for LGBT Patients in Dermatology Clinics

Justin L. Jia, BS[1], Danielle J. Polin, BA[1], Kavita Y. Sarin, MD, PhD*

KEYWORDS

- Dermatology • Organizational change • Clinic change • Lesbian • Gay • Bisexual • Transgender
- LGBT • Health disparities

KEY POINTS

- Implementing organizational and institutional change on the level of individual health care facilities can improve dermatologic care for LGBT patients.
- A clinic's workflow, staff composition, and visual cues that take a variety of forms all influence a patient's visit before they ever interact with a dermatologist.
- The clinic's physical layout and how information moves among staff affects patients' experiences during the visit and can be improved for higher-quality dermatology care.
- Improved organizational factors can make patients feel more comfortable disclosing necessary health-relevant information about themselves, such as their sexual orientation and gender identity.
- Better experiences in health care settings can increase professional care use and improve dermatology outcomes for LGBT patient populations.

INTRODUCTION

Lesbian, gay, bisexual, and transgender (LGBT) patient populations face significant health disparities—a recent national survey found that 19% of LGBT patients are denied care because of their gender identities and 28% have been harassed in health care settings.[1] This population similarly faces disproportionate risk of dermatologically relevant diseases, such as HIV, syphilis, chlamydia, genital herpes, and human papillomavirus (HPV). Previous literature finds that men who have sex with men (MSM) represented 70% of newly diagnosed HIV patients in the United States in 2014, 81% of all male cases of syphilis in 2016, and are infected with gonorrhea and chlamydia, genital herpes, and HPV at higher rates than their non-MSM counterparts.[2,3] There is less research on women who have sex with women (WSW), but some studies show that WSW exhibit higher rates of chlamydia, herpes simplex virus-2 seropositivity, bacterial vaginosis, and HPV infections than their heterosexual counterparts,[2] and are less likely to seek preventative care.[4] In addition, transgender men and women often experience unmet dermatology needs especially during gender-transition surgery,[1] implying a lack of provider knowledge about transgender-specific conditions and surgery complications. Given this systematically higher prevalence of several infectious and noninfectious dermatologic conditions among LGBT populations, it is important to understand what drives these disparities, and how clinical spaces can be improved to mitigate them.

Department of Dermatology, Stanford University School of Medicine, 455 Broadway Street, MC 8843, Redwood City, CA 94063, USA
[1] Authors contributed equally.
* Corresponding author.
E-mail address: ksarin@stanford.edu

Dermatol Clin 38 (2020) 269–276
https://doi.org/10.1016/j.det.2019.10.012
0733-8635/20/© 2019 Elsevier Inc. All rights reserved.

derm.theclinics.com

Many factors are thought to contribute to the perpetuation of disparities in health care for LGBT patients. Among the possible contributors is that health care professionals often lack the training to encourage patients to disclose their sexual orientation in a culturally sensitive manner[4]; in fact, the knowledge gap is so significant that a 2016 survey of oncologists found that only 28% of responders felt themselves to be well-informed on the health needs of the LGBT population.[5] A lack of cultural competence on behalf of health care providers and supporting clinical staff can have a detrimental effect on the patient-doctor relationship. The mistrust it can breed prevents successful and productive communication between patient and provider, and negatively affects patient compliance with their prescribed treatment regimens.[6] As the patient-doctor relationship is particularly important in determining a patient's future use of health care, LGBT patients are comparatively more likely to avoid or delay seeking professional health care services.[6] This avoidance exacerbates the disparity in disease prevalence, as clinical encounters are necessary for prevention, screening, and treatment. However, although the patient-doctor relationship is vital, and has been studied extensively in previous research, there are underlying organizational drivers that affect that relationship and patients' other interactions within professional health care, especially within dermatology, an outpatient oriented and specialized medical field. Because the structure and operations of a facility are such a significant part of a patient's visit, optimizing those factors is a vital precursor to be addressed in improving quality of care and dermatologic health outcomes for this population. Building on practice change literature,[7–9] this paper focuses on 5 domains of organizational operations that can be used to improve dermatologic care for LGBT people: clinic workflow and operations, emerging technologies and electronic health records (EHRs), clinic culture, clinic environment and resource availability, and provider and staff education (Fig. 1).

Clinic Workflow and Operations

The workflow and operations of a clinic can be defined as how patients, staff, and information move through a clinic, and how tasks are shared and completed throughout the patient care process. They are routine and outline how various clinical staff satisfy their individual roles in the larger scheme of successful patient care. Thoughtfully designed and clearly

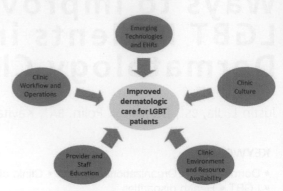

Fig. 1. Domains for Improving Care for LGBT Patients in the Dermatology Clinic.

defined workflows can lessen the activation energy required for integrating components of culturally sensitive care into every patient visit, leading to higher standards for care and inclusivity.

There are several key components of a clinic's workflow and operations that influence patient experiences, and especially the experience of LGBT patients who may expect discrimination from providers or otherwise negative experiences based on lived experience or the experience of peers or reference groups.[6] Patient flow through clinic, the workflow that the care team uses to move through a patient's tasks as well as between patients, and the composition of the care team itself are all aspects of a patient's visit to a dermatology clinic that tremendously influence their experience. Such modalities can be optimized to improve a patient's experience when seeking dermatologic care.

Patient pre-encounter experience

On entering the clinic and checking in for an appointment, it is standard to have first-time patients fill out intake questionnaires used for screening purposes. Typically, questions related to demographics, sun-exposure, skin cancer risk, and other cutaneous conditions are asked. Assuring that the demographic questions in these questionnaires use inclusive language is a relatively low-resource way to immediately create a safe and welcoming environment for LGBT patients. For example, offering a variety of answer options for questions asking for the patient's preferred gender and title, or formatting the answer spaces to be open-ended rather than multiple choice, can signal to the patient that the clinic is sensitive to such questions and respectful of all identities.

Questionnaires can also include questions related to sexual habits and sexually transmitted infections. It is generally easier to reveal personal information on paper than it is to another person, and because LGBT patients may expect discrimination in response to their answers, the difficulty of revealing that information about themselves may be especially mitigated through depersonalized methods. Encouraging disclosure of sexual orientation and gender identity in a comfortable way is highly beneficial for the patient and for the clinic; information about a patient's sexual orientation and gender identity can lead to improved access to professional care, the quality of that care by informing the physician as to the patient's predisposed dermatologic risks, and ultimately health outcomes.[10–13]

The clinic's repertoire of paper-based resources that are housed in the waiting room can also be expanded to include culturally sensitive resources specific to LGBT populations, such as community guides, tip sheets, or tailored materials that, for example, detail different skin cancer risks among sexual minorities. Their presence may also serve as a physical cue of a welcoming environment, encouraging patient trust from the onset.

On being called out of the waiting room, a pivotal point of a culturally sensitive clinic workflow is being aware of the name and pronoun by which the patient prefers to be addressed. For example, many transgender people do not go by their legal name. Regardless of intention, mis-gendering an individual or calling them by a name that they have chosen not to identify with at best invalidates an identity and at worst is triggering and can preemptively deter any trust-building between the patient and their care team.

Clinical staff flow through patient tasks and between patients

Strong communication among staff members is crucial for functional clinic workflow but is especially important for a clinic that sees LGBT patients. Without effective communication between care team members, heteronormative assumptions may accidently be made. Heteronormative language and assumptions can make patients uncomfortable,[14] and have been shown to deter LGBT patients from disclosing information about themselves that may be relevant to their health—a 2016 study found that exposure to heteronormative language makes LGBT patients about 30% less likely to disclose their sexual health to a provider relative to peers who were exposed to more inclusive language.[15] This lack of disclosure contributes to poorer health outcomes than in the case of their counterparts who are comfortable disclosing, discussing, and receiving professional

input about all of their medical concerns. Effective communication is therefore required as the patient is handed off between care team members to ensure that patients are not burdened with having to reaffirm their identity anew in each interaction, or made to feel uncomfortable and thus less likely to engage fully with the subsequent encounter.

Between patients, it is important to review their charts and to ensure that the preferred name and pronoun is being used. An innocent slip of the tongue or a brief confusion with a previous patient may be interpreted as insensitive. If such a mistake does happen during the clinical encounter, it is important that the provider pause, acknowledge their mistake, and correct themselves in future statements. Small gestures, such as this can positively affect patient-doctor trust and communication.

Care team composition

A care team that works well together and has an implemented structure has been shown to decrease burnout among the staff members.[16] Less burnout allows for more efficient work, fewer mistakes, and a higher capacity for full and careful engagement with each patient care task. These factors combine to facilitate higher-quality care, so it is worth thoughtfully composing a team that would work well together and communicate effectively.

In addition to strong and positive team dynamics, a diverse care team offers a patient a wider perspective and a more widely informed pool of knowledge among the patient's health care advocates. Literature shows that the patient-provider interaction is improved when the patient can personally relate with their provider—previous research finds that patients are 0.19 times more likely to trust their physician, 0.18 times more likely to be satisfied with their care, and 0.31 times more likely to adhere to their treatment regimen if they perceive themselves to be similar to their physician.[17] Therefore, given the diversity of patients at a given clinic, it is best practice to compose diverse care teams to best suit the needs of a wide range of patients. It can be a conscious effort in the hiring process that diversity of perspectives and experiences is taken into consideration for the betterment of the care team and patients.

Electronic Health Records and Emerging Technologies

Emerging technology is revolutionizing the health care landscape by allowing users to view and share unprecedented amounts of health information at record speeds.[18] Health information technology, such as EHRs, visit notes, and patient portals facilitate an efficient transfer of information about patients' health between patients and their health care providers as well as among the rest of the clinical staff.

Similarly, social media offers a patient-centered and dynamic platform on which patients and health care professionals alike can interact outside of the traditional clinic space, where there may be more rigid codes of conduct, and a lesser ability to share multimedia, such as videos and photos. In addition to its potential education benefits, social media can have the benefit of offering a support group for patients with similar symptoms or experiences.

Electronic health records, patient portals, and shared visit notes

Because LGBT status is often not outwardly apparent, it may be helpful to allow patients to describe their gender and sexual orientation in the EHR.[19] This mechanism of disclosure would offer similar privacy as the paper-based intake form filled out on the first visit to a clinic, with the additional benefit of the patient being able to fill it out on their own time and in the comfort of their own space. As with the paper-based questionnaire, this strategy could benefit the entire clinic population, but because LGBT patients may expect discrimination in response to their answers, this private mechanism may further encourage disclosure.

Sharing visit notes among clinic staff ensures a patient not needing to repeat personal information. Especially when the repetition concerns their identities or sensitive information that is difficult to discuss repeatedly, the patient's comfort might be challenged with excessive repetition of sensitive information. LGBT patients report that providers often seem to lack knowledge about LGBT-specific dermatologic health issues,[3,19] and so it vital to avoid placing the burden of educating individual care team members on the patient. Similarly, it is worth recognizing that it may be burdensome for the patient to come in and discuss difficult topics with their provider, so sharing notes between care team members prevents the emotional discomfort of having to summon the effort anew.

Social media

As a increasing number of adults nationwide are engaging in social media,[20] and a sizable portion of them are using it to access health-related information,[21] social media is a powerful resource for clinic staff to use to engage and empower their patients. Sixty-five percent of physicians use social media for professional purposes,[22] and can take advantage of its broad reach to contact LGBT communities to more personally address specific concerns or reservations about their clinic or the aspect of seeking care.

Similarly, some hospitals and clinics support disease-specific Facebook groups that patients can use to discuss shared experiences, exchange recommendations, or simply receive and/or offer a sympathetic ear. For example, "The Celiac Support Group at Boston Children's Hospital" is a Facebook group run out of the Boston Children's Hospital that self-describes itself as "a community of support, education and advocacy for families with children diagnosed with celiac disease."[23] Similarly, Massachusetts General Hospital runs a Facebook group called "MGH LGBT Employee Resource Group," which serves as an educational resource to the MGH community about LGBT health.[24] Online forums offer the same benefits, also with the capability of efficient transfer of multimedia content, such as videos and photos. This low-stakes and oftentimes anonymous engagement with health information is likely to benefit LGBT patients who may otherwise not feel empowered enough to seek the same information in a physical clinic or need the additional encouragement to seek it out. Dermatology is a specialty that would especially benefit from these support groups, as symptoms are often visible and the discussion of them is well facilitated by multimedia that is easily shared online.

Clinic Culture

The displayed commitment of leadership and staff to equitable care, the diversity of the clinic workforce, and clinic referral networks are often facilitators to improving care and should be explored in the present consideration of providing cultural competent care for LGBT patients.

Staff commitment

Team-wide commitment to a mission is crucial for an organization to succeed. On a precursory level, part of the staff hiring process can include an assessment of bias and screening for the desire to work in an LGBT-friendly space. Among existing staff and leadership, it is important to ensure uniform training so that all those who interact with patients are aware of the competencies expected of them. Providers who feel comfortable doing so can also wear self-identifiers with pronouns, which may empower patients to share their own, and serve as another visual cue of inclusivity. Pronouns worn on an article of clothing signals the idea that gender identity is not necessarily outwardly apparent, which is a tenant of cultural competence that such a small act can signify to patients.

Composition of clinical and nonclinical workforce

In addition to the previously discussed benefits of diverse patient care teams, a diverse clinic workforce serves as another visual indicator of inclusivity to patients, even if not all of the visible workforce is directly involved in their care. This should be considered in the clinic staff hiring process, as a diversity of experience and perspective is beneficial both to individual patients' care and to the clinic's stated mission.

Clinic referrals networks

Given the nature of dermatology as a medical specialty, many patients find themselves at a dermatology clinic because of a referral from their primary care provider. By reaching out to local primary care providers and other physicians, clinics can make themselves known as a safe and culturally sensitive practice that prioritizes the well-being of their LGBT patients. This can create a broader network of LGBT-sensitive providers, which can in turn mitigate the struggle that LGBT patients navigating the field, either spending a disproportionately large amount of time and resources on trial-and-error or having negative care experiences and poor health outcomes as a result.

Environment and Resources

A clinic needs resources to successfully engage a diverse patient population in their health care and the decision making involved in it. Beyond the availability of resources, such as paper- and media-based educational materials, a clinic's physical environment plays a key role in facilitating trust and a positive interaction between patients and staff. Visual cues that imply a nondiscriminatory environment and the physical space to ensure patient privacy are vital in the optimization of an institutional structure to enable higher-quality dermatologic health care.

Educational materials

Because LGBT patients are subject to different risk factors for various dermatologic conditions from their nonminority counterparts, tailored educational materials must be offered to support their health care autonomy and education. For example, LGBT patients are more likely to use indoor sun-tanning. National surveys found that indoor tanning use is 2 to 6 times more likely among LGBT men than in heterosexual men, and it follows naturally that the same population was twice as likely to have reported having nonmelanoma skin cancer between 2001 and 2013.[25,26] Thus, materials that are curated for LGBT patients may help to discourage indoor sun-tanning use. Providing more relevant information has the dual purpose of more powerfully informing discussions with providers around health care options and decisions, as well as serving as a sign that the clinic is a nondiscriminatory space in which LGBT patients are welcome.

Visual cues

Previous research has shown that visual cues of a welcome and safe environment, such as gender-neutral bathroom signs, or posters showing same-sex couples or transgender people, make LGBT patients more comfortable disclosing their sexual orientation to their health care providers.[27] Visual cues are a nonconfrontational way to encourage trust in patients who may be hesitant to pursue professional dermatology care at all, and so are an efficient and effective means of preemptively shaping a positive health care experience.

Privacy

Confidentiality of information exchange between patients and their providers is standard practice, and patients should be informed of who has access to their medical information. Beyond that, however, a clinic must have the physical space for private conversations to make patients feel more comfortable disclosing their identities, discussing sexual practices, and bringing up health concerns. Feelings of vulnerability, coupled with possible past experiences of discrimination or even violence, could make dermatology visits especially difficult for LGBT patients. For this reason, it is vital to verbally and physically ensure privacy to all patients by providing private examination rooms, curtains to block parts of the room from sight in case the door were to open, and a structure in which conversations cannot be overheard. Physical vulnerability is especially relevant to dermatology, where showing skin lesions to a health care provider often necessitates the removal of items of clothing.

Avoiding professional dermatology care for fear of discrimination or extreme vulnerability can have detrimental effects on a patient's health. For example, it has been found that transgender women prefer to have their face changed, for which noninvasive options include neurotoxin injections, cosmetic filler injections, or laser hair removal are available, before having their sexual organs changed,.[28,29] Previously, transgender women would regularly attempt to obtain these filler injections through illegal means or from nonmedical personnel, which curtails safe use, follow-up, and even confirmation of the safety of the filler injection itself.[28,30,31] There have been several cases of granulomatous reactions, lymphatic and vascular compromise, and even death as a result of these illicit practices.[30] Thus, whereas many procedures may be cosmetic in nature, avoidance of professional care to obtain those procedures can have disastrous consequences, and it is important to provide patients with a safe and private space in which to share what they want from their care.

Provider and Staff Education

Education and training are necessary for all levels of staff who interact with patients and has been shown to improve cultural competence in clinical interaction.[32] There are currently few curricula in place as part of standard health care training that emphasize cultural competency specific to LGBT patients, and ongoing education is even rarer.[33] Patient identities and their dermatology needs are continuously morphing alongside a changing health care landscape, which includes an increasingly interconnected world, an evolving definition of community that is no longer confined to physical proximity, and a growing national platform for the discussion of sexual and gender identity issues. Therefore, it is vital to start education about LGBT issues in dermatology as early as residency training, to implement medical continuing education with respect to them, and to use cultural humility training for dermatologic staff in clinics.

Residency training and education
For many practicing dermatologists, residency often is one of the final stages of medical training. The knowledge and skills that one builds in residency form the foundation for life-long clinical practice. Residency training, thus, is an opportune time to teach LGBT-focused curricular content, and train dermatologists how to provide appropriate culturally sensitive care (**Table 1**). In addition, best-practices such as the use of intake forms to gather sexual orientation and gender identity data may also be incorporated into residency teaching, as there is often a lack of training surrounding how to incorporate such operations to improve patient experiences. Clinics can also look to hire from programs with known LGBT content in their residency curricula or implement strong post-schooling training programs to ensure high-quality care for their LGBT patients.

Continuing medical education
Given the rarity of the inclusion of so many key aspects of LGBT care in dermatology curricula, additional training and education at the post-schooling level is vital for providers and other staff members who interact with patients. Health care organizations can use existing tools, such as the Healthcare Equality Index,[35] to determine their current competence for LGBT patients and encourage provider participation in continuing medical education so they can be abreast with the latest treatment options. Supplementing and providing resources for providers to participate in these workshops would hugely benefit the aspects of care that are lacking due to knowledge or training gaps.

Cultural humility training for clinic staff
In addition to training about specific aspects of dermatology that are relevant to the health of LGBT patients and the health disparities that affect this population, it is also important for providers and clinical staff to train and have ongoing discussions around cultural competency and humility. This kind of training requires more than facts, but rather a practice of attitude and empathy. All health care providers have committed to lifelong learning, and understanding their patient's identities and cultures in their own context and nonjudgmentally is part of that commitment to the medical community.

SUMMARY

The organizational and institutional operations of dermatology clinics shape the context of every interaction a patient has in that clinic. These operations set the tone for a visit and provide its background throughout. Although the actual interactions that a patient has with clinical staff and dermatology providers are the points at which health care occurs, they are immeasurably influenced by the experience that a patient has in the clinic before ever speaking with that health care professional as well as by the physical space in which that interaction occurs. Thus, by focusing on and optimizing clinic workflow, EHRs, organizational structure, environment, community engagement, and education for clinical staff to provide higher quality care for LGBT patients, dermatology clinics will be better able to serve this population and mitigate the significant disparities it presently faces.

DISCLOSURE

The authors have nothing to disclose.

Table 1
Potential LGBT-focused curricular topics for dermatology residencies

Curriculum Content	Description and Sample Topics
Dermatologic conditions secondary to HIV/AIDS	Those infected with HIV/AIDS are much more susceptible to conditions, such as Kaposi sarcoma, molluscum contagiosum, and photodermatitis because of the weakened immunity associated with the virus.
Pronoun use and identifiers for LGBT patients	Introducing oneself with their pronouns both creates the opportunity for patients to do the same, and signals the understanding that gender is not necessarily outwardly apparent, indicating respect and empathy toward a patient's identities.
Skin cancer risk among sexual minority men and women	As previously discussed, sexual and/or gender minority people have a higher risk of skin cancer than their heterosexual counterparts due largely to higher indoor tanning use. Educating health providers about these different risk factors may improve preventative medicine for LGBT patients, or inform providers about screening they should be considering.
Injectable/neurotoxin and filler for facial modification in transitioning patients	The use of illicit or otherwise subpar injections can lead to a host of complications ranging in severity and must be screened for by providers. A detailed history, conducted in a culturally sensitive manner, can elucidate previous soft tissue injections or risk factors for their use.
Effects of hormone therapy and gender-confirming surgeries on skin and hair of transitioning patients	There are many potential complications and necessary considerations in gender-confirming surgeries. For example, patients undergoing "bottom surgery" may require laser hair removal, and in transgender women, intravaginal hair can cause discomfort or infection.[2] In addition, alopecia may develop in transgender men as a result of testosterone treatment,[2] something that a dermatologist should discuss with patients.
LGBT oriented history taking and physical exam	In addition to previously described considerations of sensitively asking for sexual orientation and gender identity, there are unique considerations in physical exam taking for transgender patients. In transgender women, the neovagina differs from a natal vagina, and the use of an anoscope may be more appropriate for a visual exam.[34] In transgender men, it is important to keep in mind that a pelvic exam may induce anxiety, and so it is important not to subject the patient to more exams than are necessary. Chest binding and tucking of testicles and the penis are additional considerations in culturally sensitive physical exam taking.[34]

REFERENCES

1. Yeung H, Luk KM, Chen SC, et al. Dermatologic care for lesbian, gay, bisexual, and transgender persons: terminology, demographics, health disparities, and approaches to care. J Am Acad Dermatol 2019; 80(3):581–9.

2. Yeung H, Luk KM, Chen SC, et al. Dermatologic care for lesbian, gay, bisexual, and transgender persons: epidemiology, screening, and disease prevention. J Am Acad Dermatol 2019;80(3):591–602.

3. Lesbian, gay, bisexual, and transgender health | healthy people 2020. Available at: https:// www.healthypeople.gov/2020/topics-objectives/topic/ lesbian-gay-bisexual-and-transgender-health. Accessed April 5, 2019.

4. DeMeester RH, Lopez FY, Moore JE, et al. A model of organizational context and shared decision making: application to LGBT racial and ethnic minority patients. J Gen Intern Med 2016;31(6):651–62.

5. Shetty G, Sanchez JA, Lancaster JM, et al. Oncology healthcare providers' knowledge, attitudes, and practice behaviors regarding LGBT health. Patient Educ Couns 2016;99(10): 1676–84.

6. Chin MH, Lopez FY, Nathan AG, et al. Improving shared decision making with LGBT racial and ethnic minority patients. J Gen Intern Med 2016;31(6):591–3.

7. Eckstrand KL, Lunn MR, Yehia BR. Applying Organizational Change to Promote Lesbian, Gay, Bisexual, and Transgender Inclusion and Reduce Health Disparities. LGBT Health 2017;4(3):174–80.

8. Kauth MR, Shipherd JC. Transforming a System: Improving Patient-Centered Care for Sexual and Gender Minority Veterans. LGBT Health 2016;3(3): 177–9.

9. Demeester RH, Lopez FY, Moore JE, et al. A Model of Organizational Context and Shared Decision Making: Application to LGBT Racial and Ethnic Minority Patients. Journal of General Internal Medicine 2016;31(6):651–62.

10. Cahill S, Makadon H. Sexual orientation and gender identity data collection in clinical settings and in electronic health records: a key to ending LGBT health disparities. LGBT Health 2013;1(1):34–41.

11. Kamen CS, Smith-Stoner M, Heckler CE, et al. Social support, self-rated health, and lesbian, gay, bisexual, and transgender identity disclosure to cancer care providers. Oncol Nurs Forum 2015;42(1):44–51.

12. Gao Y, Katz KA. Clinical and serologic evolution of multiple penile chancres in a man who has sex with men. JAMA Dermatol 2018;154(1):108–9.

13. Birkhäuer J, Gaab J, Kossowsky J, et al. Trust in the health care professional and health outcome: a meta-analysis. PLoS One 2017;12(2):e0170988.

14. Charny JW, Kovarik CL. LGBT access to health care: a dermatologist's role in building a therapeutic relationship. Cutis 2017;99(4):228–9.

15. Utamsingh PD, Richman LS, Martin JL, et al. Heteronormativity and practitioner-patient interaction. Health Commun 2016;31(5):566–74.

16. Willard-Grace R, Hessler D, Rogers E, et al. Team structure and culture are associated with lower burnout in primary care. J Am Board Fam Med 2014;27(2):229–38.

17. Street RL, O'Malley KJ, Cooper LA, et al. Understanding concordance in patient-physician relationships: personal and ethnic dimensions of shared identity. Ann Fam Med 2008;6(3):198–205.

18. Jia JL, Polin DJ, Sarin KY. Emerging Technologies for Health Information in Dermatology: Opportunities and Drawbacks of Web-based Searches, Social Media, Mobile Applications, and Direct-to-Consumer Genetic Testing in Patient Care. Sem Cutan Med Surg 2019;38(1):E57–63.

19. Mansh MD, Nguyen A, Katz KA. Improving dermatologic care for sexual and gender minority patients through routine sexual orientation and gender identity data collection. JAMA Dermatol 2018. https://doi.org/10.1001/jamadermatol.2018.3909.

20. Demographics of social media users and adoption in the United States. Available at: https://www.pewinternet.org/fact-sheet/social-media/. Accessed April 5, 2019.

21. PricewaterhouseCoopers. Social media "likes" healthcare: From marketing to social business. PwC. Available at: https://www.pwc.com/us/en/health-industries/health-research-institute/publications/health-care-social-media.html. Accessed October 3, 2018.

22. Ventola CL. Social media and health care professionals: benefits, risks, and best practices. P T 2014;39(7):491–520.

23. Celiac kids connection at Boston Children's Hospital—About. Available at: https://www.facebook.com/pg/ChildrensCeliac/about/. Accessed April 5, 2019.

24. MGH LGBT employee resource group - about. Available at: https://www.facebook.com/pg/MGHLGBT/about/?ref=page_internal. Accessed April 5, 2019.

25. Yeung H, Chen SC. Sexual orientation and indoor tanning device use: a population-based study. JAMA Dermatol 2016;152(1):99–101.

26. Mansh M, Katz KA, Linos E, et al. Association of skin cancer and indoor tanning in sexual minority men and women. JAMA Dermatol 2015;151(12):1308–16.

27. Guidelines for care of lesbian, gay, bisexual, and transgender patients | National Prevention Information Network. Available at: https://npin.cdc.gov/publication/guidelines-care-lesbian-gay-bisexual-and-transgender-patients. Accessed April 5, 2019.

28. Sullivan P, Trinidad J, Hamann D. Issues in transgender dermatology: a systematic review of the literature. J Am Acad Dermatol 2019. https://doi.org/10.1016/j.jaad.2019.03.023.

29. Ginsberg BA, Calderon M, Seminara NM, et al. A potential role for the dermatologist in the physical transformation of transgender people: a survey of attitudes and practices within the transgender community. J Am Acad Dermatol 2016;74(2):303–8.

30. Ginsberg BA. Dermatologic care of the transgender patient. Int J Womens Dermatol 2017;3(1):65–7.

31. Marks DH, Awosika O, Rengifo-Pardo M, et al. Dermatologic surgical care for transgender individuals. Dermatol Surg 2019;45(3):446–57.

32. Delgado DA, Ness S, Ferguson K, et al. Cultural competence training for clinical staff: measuring the effect of a one-hour class on cultural competence. J Transcult Nurs 2013;24(2):204–13.

33. Park AJ, Katz KA. Paucity of lesbian, gay, bisexual, and transgender health-related content in the basic dermatology curriculum. JAMA Dermatol 2018;154(5):614–5.

34. Guidelines for the primary and gender-affirming care of transgender and gender nonbinary people: transgender patients and the physical examination. Available at: http://transhealth.ucsf.edu/trans?page=guidelines-physical-examination. Accessed April 5, 2019.

35. Healthcare Equality Index 2018 | human rights campaign. Available at: https://www.hrc.org/hei. Accessed April 5, 2019.

Trainee Exposure and Education for Minimally Invasive Gender-Affirming Procedures

Brittany Buhalog, MD[a],*, Jon Klint Peebles, MD[b], Matthew Mansh, MD[c],
Esther A. Kim, MD[d], Philip Daniel Knott, MD[e], William Hoffman, MD[d],
Rahul Seth, MD[f], Andre Alcon, MD[d], Sarah Tuttleton Arron, MD, PhD[g]

KEYWORDS

- Transgender • Medical education • Minimally invasive procedures • Gender-affirming procedures
- Cultural humility • Nonbinary

KEY POINTS

- Minimally invasive gender-affirmation procedures (MIGAPs) align gender identity and expression in a manner that is effective, safe, and reversible to accommodate the needs of a variety of gender-nonbinary or transgender patients.
- Soft tissue augmentation, laser hair removal, and neuromodulator injections are performed by dermatology residents and fellows. Soft tissue augmentation and body contouring procedures are performed by nondermatology procedural trainees.
- Specific education regarding the safe and effective use of MIGAPs was provided in a minority of polled programs.
- Didactic teaching sessions, formal faculty demonstrations on planned patients, organic trainee observation in clinic, and staff supervision of residents/fellows performing the procedures were the most commonly used methods of MIGAP education.

INTRODUCTION

There are more than 1 million transgender and gender-nonbinary individuals living in the United States.[1] This population has unique health care needs, is largely marginalized in the current health care system, and is historically excluded from research. Many gender minority individuals seek gender-affirming surgical procedures to better align their physical appearance with their gender identity. Gender-affirming procedures, including so-called top and bottom surgeries, have been shown to improve quality of life and psychological well-being.[2,3] For example, facial feminization procedures for gender affirmation include brow lifting, hairline advancement, rhinoplasty, facelifting, jaw

[a] UCSF Dermatologic surgery and laser center: 1701 Divisadero St, San Francisco, CA 94115, USA; [b] Department of Dermatology, Kaiser Permanente Mid-Atlantic Permanente Medical Group, Rockville, MD, USA; [c] Department of Dermatology, University of Minnesota School of Medicine, Minneapolis, MN, USA; [d] Division of Plastic and Reconstructive Surgery, University of California, San Francisco, San Francisco, CA, USA; [e] Section of Facial Plastic Surgery, Facial Plastic and Reconstructive Surgery, Department of Otolaryngology/Head and Neck Surgery, UCSF Medical Center, San Francisco, CA, USA; [f] Facial Plastic and Reconstructive Surgery, UCSF Department of Otolaryngology- Head and Neck Surgery (OHNS), San Francisco, CA, USA; [g] San Francisco VA Medical Center, UCSF Dermatologic Surgery and Laser Center, San Francisco, CA, USA
* Corresponding author.
E-mail address: bbuhalog@gmail.com

Dermatol Clin 38 (2020) 277–283
https://doi.org/10.1016/j.det.2019.10.009
0733-8635/20/© 2019 Elsevier Inc. All rights reserved.

and tracheal reduction, and cheek implants or fat grafting. Less attention has been given to the role of minimally invasive gender-affirming procedures (MIGAPs) in the care of this population, particularly for those patients who are preparing for more invasive procedures. MIGAPs, which include laser hair removal, neuromodulators, and soft tissue augmentation, may be options for those individuals seeking less invasive, nonpermanent or semipermanent gender affirmation (**Table 1**). It is important that providers are adequately trained to provide this care.

Initial research suggests that graduate medical education (GME) curricula may lack content related to transgender and gender-affirming care. Trainees in plastic surgery, oral and maxillofacial surgery, and urologic surgery receive only a few hours annually of education focused on

gender-affirming surgery,[4–6] and trainees in family medicine, psychiatry, and endocrinology report limited education and lack of preparedness for caring for the transgender population.[7] No studies, to our knowledge, have attempted to ascertain the amount and type of GME dedicated specifically to MIGAPs. This study assessed the prevalence, extent, and types of clinical exposure and formal curricular education related to MIGAPs among GME training programs in specialties that routinely perform minimally invasive surgical procedures.

MATERIALS AND METHODS
Survey Design

A brief survey was designed by study investigators using the REDCap (Research Electronic Data Capture) online survey platform to assess current

Table 1
Effects and considerations of minimally invasive gender-affirming procedures

Procedure	Effect	Risks	Comments
Neuromodulators	• Change brow position and arch • Reduce masseter bulk to contour or slim the jawline	• Ptosis • Bruising • Facial asymmetry	• Temporary effects; excellent for patients with fluid gender identities who wish to alter expression frequently • Masseter bulk reduction can be more sustained
Soft tissue augmentation	• Increase forehead projection • Contour jawline • Augment lip fullness • Alter malar cheek projection • Enhance chin projection • Enhance tracheal projection or create an Adam's apple	• Intravascular injection • Granulomatous inflammatory response • Infection • Blindness • Soft tissue necrosis • Facial asymmetry	• Hyaluronic acid is dissolvable and semi-permanent, and can be reversed easily to accommodate patients with fluid gender identity • Gradual changes in appearances permissible over time • Silicone injections offer permanent results, but complications are difficult to manage
Body contouring	• Redistribution of subcutaneous fat to abdomen or buttocks/thighs	• Fluid shifts with liposuction • Bruising, hematoma, swelling • Intravascular injection of deoxycholate could lead to skin necrosis	• Longer downtime postprocedure
Laser or light-based devices	• After gender-affirming surgical scar revision • Hair removal • Nonmedicinal acne treatment	- Hyperpigmentation/hypopigmentation, blistering, bruising, infection, pain	• Effects can be permanent or irreversible

education for MIGAPs in core surgical and procedural programs. The survey consisted of 7 items estimated to require 5 minutes or less, and was designed to be easily administered on a mobile device. Questions were modeled after similar surveys in the literature.[7–10] This study qualified as quality assessment, and thus was considered Institutional Review Board exempt in the authors' institutions. shows a copy of the disseminated survey.

Participants

All current program directors (PDs) for core surgical and procedural residency and fellowship training programs (cosmetic dermatology, aesthetic plastic surgery, oculoplastic and reconstructive surgery, Mohs micrographic surgery, integrated plastic surgery, otolaryngology, and dermatology) were considered for study participation. Exclusion criteria included the inability to obtain an e-mail address and no involvement of trainees in minimally invasive cosmetic procedures.

Survey Dissemination

PD e-mails were obtained from online records of residency and/or fellowship governing bodies, including the Accreditation Council for Graduate Medical Education, American Society of Dermatologic Surgery, American Society for Oculoplastic and Reconstructive Surgery, American Society of Aesthetic Plastic Surgeons, and San Francisco Match Web sites. Several program coordinators were listed as points of contact for training programs rather than the PD and an e-mail was sent to the coordinator with instructions to forward to the PD. If a PD was the director of more than 1 fellowship

and/or residency program, we asked that multiple surveys be completed, 1 for each program directed.

STATISTICAL ANALYSIS

All data aggregation and analysis was performed using Microsoft Excel software.

RESULTS
Respondent and Program Demographics

The survey identified 577 core procedural and surgical fellowship and/or residency PDs, of which 527 had available e-mail addresses and therefore were eligible to participate in the survey. Of 47 survey respondents (9% response rate), 6 were excluded because of trainees not participating in minimally invasive aesthetic surgical procedures and 3 because of incomplete submitted surveys, yielding a final study sample of 38 GME programs (**Fig. 1**). Three invitations were sent over the course of 3 weeks to maximize survey response.

Most respondents were dermatology PDs (N = 22, 57.9%), which included Mohs micrographic surgery (N = 3, 8%) and cosmetic dermatology fellowship programs (N = 1, 2.6%). The remaining specialties represented included plastic surgery residency and fellowship programs (which included aesthetic plastic surgery and integrated plastic surgery; N = 9 in total, 23.7%), oculoplastic surgery (N = 1, 2.6%), and otolaryngology (N = 6, 15.8%). Most respondent PDs practiced in an academic setting. Geographic location and number of teaching physicians involved in resident or fellow education was diverse, although many programs indicated large numbers of affiliated faculty (**Table 2**). Demographics of PDs whose trainees participated in MIGAPs were similar to the demographics of overall respondents (**Table 3**).

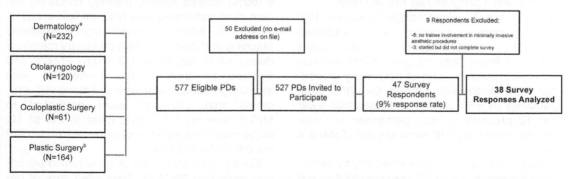

Fig. 1. Study participant selection: 577 PDs were identified in 8 core minimally invasive procedural specialties. E-mail addresses were available for 527 and these were therefore eligible for study participation. Forty-seven responded to the survey (9% response rate). Six were ultimately excluded because of lack of trainee participation in minimally invasive aesthetic procedures, and 3 failed to complete the survey. Thus, 38 responses were analyzed for this survey. [a] Included dermatology residency programs, Mohs micrographic surgery, and cosmetic dermatology fellowship programs. [b] Included plastic surgery residency programs, aesthetic plastic surgery fellowship programs, and integrated plastic surgery residency programs.

Table 2
Demographics of all responding program directors

Characteristic	All Participants (N = 38) N (%)	Dermatology[a] (N = 22) N (%)	All Others (N = 16) N (%)
Region			
West	5 (13.2)	3 (13.6)	2 (12.5)
Southwest	5 (13.2)	4 (18.2)	1 (6.3)
Midwest	10 (26.3)	5 (22.7)	4 (25.0)
Southeast	8 (21.1)	3 (13.6)	5 (31.3)
Northeast	10 (26.3)	6 (27.3)	4 (25.0)
Practice Setting			
Academic	33 (86.8)	21 (95.5)	12 (75.0)
Private practice	3 (7.9)	0 (0.0)	3 (18.8)
Unknown	2 (5.3)	1 (6.3)	1 (6.3)
Faculty Size			
<5	6 (15.8)	3 (13.6)	3 (18.8)
5–10	8 (21.1)	4 (18.2)	4 (25.0)
11–15	8 (21.1)	5 (22.7)	3 (18.8)
>15	14 (36.8)	9 (40.9)	5 (31.3)
Missing	2 (5.3)	1 (4.5)	1 (6.3)

[a] Includes cosmetic dermatology and Mohs micrographic surgery specialties.

Trainee Minimally Invasive Gender-Affirmation Procedure Clinical Exposure

Of the 38 programs that participate in minimally invasive procedures outlined earlier, 18 programs (12 dermatology programs and 6 in other specialties) indicated that trainees specifically observe or perform MIGAPs, 12 stated that their trainees did not perform these procedures, 6 were unsure whether their trainees participated (4 from otolaryngology, 1 dermatology, 1 plastic surgery), and 1 program had missing data.

Among the 12 dermatology programs that indicated trainees received clinical exposure to MIGAPs, 5 (42%) PDs reported their trainees performed fewer than 10 procedures annually and 5 (42%) were unsure of how many procedures were performed. Among the other core specialties (N = 6), 3 (50%) indicated that fewer than 10 procedures were performed annually, and the remaining half were unsure (**Tables 4** and **5**).

Laser hair removal was performed only by dermatology trainees (N = 6, 50%). Neuromodulators and soft tissue augmentation were performed by both dermatology (25.0% and 16.7%, respectively) and nondermatology (16.7% and 66.7%, respectively) trainees. Only 1 program (nondermatology) indicated that their trainees participated in body contouring procedures (see **Table 4**).

Trainee Minimally Invasive Gender-Affirmation Procedure Formal Curricular Education

Of the 18 programs that indicated that their trainees participated in MIGAPs, 10 indicated that formal education was provided during training. No programs whose trainees did not participate in MIGAPs offered education. Nine (90%) offered formal didactic education (lectures, journal clubs, small group discussions); 6 (60%) offered formal, planned hands-on patient demonstrations with resident/fellow observation; 6 (60%) provided organic bedside teaching and demonstration by faculty members during clinic hours; and 7 (70%) encouraged trainees to perform the procedures with attending/faculty supervision. Among 10 programs that provided hours dedicated to MIGAP-specific education, most (6 out of 10; 60%) spent less than 5 hours annually on MIGAP education for trainees.

Eight programs did not provide formal education regarding MIGAPs. They cited lack of patient desire (N = 2, 25%), feelings that MIGAPs require no additional training separately from minimally invasive aesthetic procedures (N = 3, 37.5%), or hoping to implement some formal education but have not yet done this (N = 3, 37.5%).

Table 3
Demographic information of programs whose trainees participate in minimally invasive gender-affirming procedures

Characteristic	No MIGAP Training[a] (N = 20) N (%)	MIGAP Training (N = 18) N (%)
Specialty		
Dermatology	10 (50.0)	12 (66.7)
All others	10 (50.0)	6 (33.3)
Region		
West	3 (15.0)	2 (11.1)
Southwest	4 (20.0)	1 (5.6)
Midwest	6 (30.0)	4 (22.2)
Southeast	2 (10.0)	6 (33.3)
Northeast	5 (25.0)	5 (27.8)
Practice Setting		
Academic	16 (80.0)	17 (94.4)
Private practice	2 (10.0)	1 (5.6)
Missing	2 (10.0)	0 (0.0)
Faculty Size		
<5	4 (20.0)	2 (11.1)
5–10	4 (20.0)	4 (22.2)
11–15	4 (20.0)	4 (22.2)
>15	6 (30.0)	8 (44.4)
Missing	2 (10.0)	0 (0.0)

[a] Indicates GME training programs that either do not include MIGAP training or in which it is unknown whether MIGAP training is included in their program.

DISCUSSION

This study highlights current deficiencies in trainee education regarding MIGAPs. Fewer than half of the responding programs provide at least some dedicated time to teaching these procedures, but those that did reported using a variety of teaching methods. The most commonly cited reason why trainees do not receive formal MIGAP education was lack of patient desire for those procedures and belief that MIGAPs do not require additional training beyond that required for adeptly performing minimally invasive procedures for purely aesthetic purposes. This finding requires further exploration but may suggest a perceived absence of bedside opportunities for education and thus a lack of necessity for formal instruction in those procedures in the surgical curriculum. Alternatively, this may indicate a lack of recognition of gender-expansive individuals and their health care needs in these communities, or, conversely, limited awareness of these procedures in gender affirmation within both the transgender patient population and their referring providers. A third possibility is patient preference to seek MIGAPs in private practice or nonacademic settings, reducing the patient demand in training programs.

MIGAPs play an important role in facilitating alignment of gender expression with gender identity. Such procedures may offer numerous advantages compared with more invasive options, including lower cost, elimination of the

Table 4
Minimally invasive gender-affirming procedures exposure per program

Characteristic	All Programs (N = 18) N (%)	Dermatology*(N = 12) N (%)	All Others (N = 6) N (%)
Annual MIGAPs Per Trainee			
<10	8 (44.4)	5 (41.7)	3 (50)
10–40	1 (5.6)	1 (8.3)	0 (0)
>40	1 (5.6)	1 (8.3)	0 (0)
Unknown	8 (44.4)	5 (41.7)	3 (50)
Types of MIGAPs Performed			
Neuromodulators	4 (22.2)	3 (25)	1 (16.7)
Soft tissue augmentation/ dermal fillers	6 (33.3)	2 (16.7)	4 (66.7)
Laser hair removal	6 (33.3)	6 (50)	0 (0)
Body contouring	1 (5.6)	0 (0)	1 (16.7)
Unknown	1 (5.6)	0 (0)	1 (16.7)

Body contouring includes tumescent liposuction, deoxycholate injections, cryolipolysis, and so forth.
* Includes dermatology residency programs, Mohs micrographic surgery, and cosmetic dermatology fellowship programs.

Table 5
Formal minimally invasive gender-affirming procedures education

Characteristic	All Programs (N = 10) N (%)	Dermatology* (N = 8) N (%)	All Others (N = 2) N (%)
Type of Education Provided			
Didactics	9 (90)	8 (100)	1 (50)
Formal faculty demonstrations	6 (60)	5 (62.5)	1 (50)
Bedside teaching	6 (60)	5 (62.5)	1 (50)
Supervision of trainees	7 (70)	6 (75)	1 (50)
Education Hours			
<1	1 (10)	0 (0)	1 (50)
1–2	4 (40)	4 (50)	0 (0)
>2–5	1 (10)	0 (0)	1 (50)
>5	4 (40)	4 (50)	0 (0)

Formal didactic sessions include lectures, journal clubs, small group discussions. Formal faculty demonstrations include formal hands-on patient demonstrations by faculty, with resident/fellow observation. Bedside teaching includes organic bedside teaching and demonstration during faculty practice. Supervision of trainee is defined as supervision of resident/fellow performing MIGAPs.
* Includes dermatology residency programs, Mohs micrographic surgery, and cosmetic dermatology fellowship programs.

need for general anesthesia, shorter recovery time, nonpermanence, and potentially greater availability and access. Although the skills necessary to perform minimally invasive procedures for aesthetic purposes may inform gender affirmation, they cannot be broadly extrapolated. Important considerations include the approach to nonbinary expression objectives when neither classically masculine nor feminine features are desired. Such concepts may not be intuitive to trainees and thus formalized education regarding leveraging these procedures to fulfill the needs of transgender and nonbinary populations is warranted. As the health care landscape becomes more welcoming to gender-expansive individuals consonant with greater visibility of this population, demand for the full range of gender-affirmation treatment options is likely to increase, highlighting the importance of meeting this anticipated need through inclusive curricula.

In terms of curricular inclusion, our results are similar to other studies investigating MIGAP curricula in other surgical or medical specialties, which indicated only a few hours dedicated to this content in a minority of polled programs.[4-7]

The importance of targeted instruction in MIGAPs for the gender-expansive population becomes readily apparent when viewed through a cultural competency lens. The concept of cultural competency in medical education emphasizes that a rudimentary understanding of minority cultures fosters more appropriate care.[11] More recently, attention has shifted to an educational paradigm of cultural humility, which stresses lifelong and longitudinal learning rooted in cultural awareness and interpersonal reflection rather than a focus on demonstrating proficiency in discrete episodes of care with an end result of competency fulfillment.[12] As such, efforts to integrate gender-expansive health into procedural curricula should blend cultural understanding with targeted procedural skill development such that trainee awareness of the needs of gender-expansive patients is not confined to the procedure.

Medical students and trainees continue to indicate that they lack preparedness for comfortably providing adequate care to this patient population.[13] Those who have frequent clinical exposure to gender minority patients have greater awareness of the unique health care needs of gender-expansive individuals and think themselves better equipped to provide appropriate care compared with those who receive only theoretic and didactic training.[14] In our study, several programs indicated that a method of teaching MIGAPs was observation or clinical experience, using bedside teaching to highlight best practices. However, data are currently lacking regarding perceived preparedness among trainees performing MIGAPs for transgender and gender-expansive patients with didactic compared with experiential education.

Although this study attempted to establish a broad survey of the current state of MIGAP education, it was limited by the low response rate. More than 500 PDs were surveyed in several disciplines, but fewer than 10% of invited participants responded. This low response rate may affect the ability to generalize our results and may not reflect education or trainee involvement in MIGAPs. It is possible that there was a bias in response to those PDs with interest in this area, which would result in an overestimation of the true exposure of trainees to MIGAPs. Additional research, including surveys of trainees, will be needed to further explore this area.

SUMMARY

This study evaluates the current landscape regarding trainee education and experience with MIGAPs in core procedural specialties. There is limited clinical exposure and education dedicated to MIGAPs during training and potentially a lack of awareness regarding the health care needs of transgender and nonbinary individuals in these communities. Further research is necessary to address these concerns, including surveys of trainee attitudes and perceptions with regard to MIGAP education as well as procedural needs assessments of the transgender and nonbinary communities to include perceived barriers to such care. Although the Accreditation Council for Graduate Medical Education (ACGME) does not yet require inclusion of transgender health content in curricula, programs should consider incorporating targeted measurement of trainee exposure to MIGAPs in their own curricula along with case log requirements.

DISCLOSURE

S.T. Arron reports the following conflicts of interest: investigator for Leo Pharma, SunPharma, Menlo Therapeutics, Castle Biosciences, Genentech/Roche, Pfizer, Regeneron, Eli Lilly, Pelle-Pharm; consultant for Enspectra Health, Regeneron, Sanofi-Genzyme, Castle Creek Pharmaceuticals, SunPharma, Pennside Partners, Biossance, Gerson Lehrman Group, Rakuten Aspyrian. The remaining authors have nothing to disclose.

REFERENCES

1. Meerwijk EL, Sevelius JM. Transgender population size in the United States: a meta-regression of population-based probability samples. Am J Public Health 2017;107(2):e1–8.

2. Defreyne J, Motmans J, T'sjoen G. Healthcare costs and quality of life outcomes following gender affirming surgery in trans men: a review. Expert Rev Pharmacoecon Outcomes Res 2017;17(6):543–56.

3. Lindqvist EK, Sigurjonsson H, Möllermark C, et al. Quality of life improves early after gender reassignment surgery in transgender women. Eur J Plast Surg 2017;40(3):223–6.

4. Dy GW, Osbun NC, Morrison SD, et al, Transgender Education Study Group. Exposure to and attitudes regarding transgender education among urology residents. J Sex Med 2016;13(10):1466–72.

5. Morrison SD, Chong HJ, Dy GW, et al. Educational exposure to transgender patient care in plastic surgery training. Plast Reconstr Surg 2016;138(4):944–53.

6. Massenburg BB, Morrison SD, Rashidi V, et al. Educational exposure to transgender patient care in otolaryngology training. J Craniofac Surg 2018; 29(5):1252–7.

7. Coutin A, Wright S, Li C, et al. Missed opportunities: are residents prepared to care for transgender patients? A study of family medicine, psychiatry, endocrinology, and urology residents. Can Med Educ J 2018;9(3):e41–55. Available at: http://www.ncbi.nlm. nih.gov/pubmed/30140346. Accessed July 27, 2018.

8. Surgeons AS of P. American Society of plastic Surgeons 2011 plastic surgery Statistics report. 2010. Available at: http://www.plasticsurgery.org/ Documents/news-resources/statistics/2011-statistics/ 2011_Stats_Full_Report.pdf.

9. Housman TS, Hancox JG, Mir MR, et al. What specialties perform the most common outpatient cosmetic procedures in the United States?: Specialties performing cosmetic procedures. Dermatol Surg 2007;34(1). https://doi.org/10.1111/j.1524-4725.2007.34000.x.

10. Heidekrueger PI, Juran S, Patel A, et al. Plastic surgery statistics in the US: evidence and implications. Aesthetic Plast Surg 2016;40(2):293–300.

11. Saha S, Beach MC, Cooper LA. Patient centeredness, cultural competence and healthcare quality. J Natl Med Assoc 2008;100(11): 1275–85.

12. Prasad SJ, Nair P, Gadhvi K, et al. Cultural humility: treating the patient, not the illness. Med Educ Online 2016;21(1):30908.

13. Korpaisarn S, Safer JD. Gaps in transgender medical education among healthcare providers: a major barrier to care for transgender persons. Rev Endocr Metab Disord 2018. https://doi.org/10.1007/s11154-018-9452-5.

14. Park JA, Safer JD. Clinical exposure to transgender medicine improves students' preparedness above levels seen with didactic teaching alone: a key addition to the boston university model for teaching transgender healthcare. Transgend Health 2018; 3(1):10–6.

Incorporating Lesbian, Gay, Bisexual, and Transgender Training into a Residency Program

Joseph W. Fakhoury, BS, Steven Daveluy, MD*

KEYWORDS

- LGBT • Cultural competence • Residency training • LGBT health • LGBT dermatology

KEY POINTS

- Incorporating lesbian, gay, bisexual, and transgender (LGBT) education into dermatology residency training can improve cultural competence and eliminate health care disparities.
- LGBT health education during residency can be improved through curricular enhancements and departmental/institutional climate optimization. Faculty with expertise in LGBT health can lead this process.
- LGBT health curricular teachings can be incorporated into the Accreditation Council on Graduate Medical Education core competencies and assessed with the dermatology milestones.
- Climate optimization occurs at the departmental or institutional level and requires competency training for all health care providers and support staff.
- LGBT-competent physicians can publicize their expertise and build a referral network for LGBT patients.

INTRODUCTION

Lesbian, gay, bisexual, and transgender (LGBT) individuals represent about 2.2% to 4% of the US population.[1] Patients who identify as LGBT individuals have insufficient access to health care services,[2,3] likely because of inadequate provider training and patients' fear of discrimination.[2,4–7]

Health care disparities (HCD) in the LGBT population include higher rates substance abuse, smoking, depression/anxiety, and violence victimization, as well as lower rates of Pap smear and mammography screening, among others.[8] Some dermatology-specific disparities include an increased risk of skin cancer in men who have sex with men (MSM),[9,10] higher rates of sexually transmitted diseases (STDs), such as human immunodeficiency virus,[11–16] and side effects of hormonal treatments (such as acne) in transgender persons during transitional treatments.[11,12,17–20] LGBT persons may face additional HCD depending on their race, ethnicity, or socioeconomic status.[21] In addition, the minority stress model, which is the concept that stigmatization results in worse health outcomes, is common in LGBT patients.[22]

Numerous public health initiatives through government and professional health organizations have attempted to address these HCD. A 2011 Institute of Medicine Report[4] addressed LGBT discrimination and the need for more robust research. The Healthy People 2020 objectives from the Department of Health of Human Services[2]

Department of Dermatology, Wayne State University School of Medicine, 18100 Oakwood Boulevard, Suite 300, Dearborn, MI 48214, USA
* Corresponding author.
E-mail address: sdaveluy@med.wayne.edu

Dermatol Clin 38 (2020) 285–292
https://doi.org/10.1016/j.det.2019.10.013

outlined the necessity of improving LGBT health, which has been reinforced by numerous organizations: the Joint Commission, American Association of Medical Colleges (AAMC), and National Institutes of Health.[23–26] Educational initiatives for health care providers regarding LGBT culture and behavioral practices can have a positive impact on patient outcomes, as highlighted by 2 cohort studies that demonstrated a reduction in high-risk behaviors among MSM following counseling by providers with specialized training.[27,28]

The most important aspect in the promotion of durable, widespread advances in LGBT health care and the elimination of disparities is the incorporation of LGBT competence in dermatology education and training. Cultural competence in residency programs not only establishes centers of excellence for LGBT care but also ensures the dissemination of competence through training future generations of dermatologists and fosters further research advances to promote health and eliminate disparities.

LESBIAN, GAY, BISEXUAL, AND TRANSGENDER EDUCATION IN MEDICAL EDUCATION

Cultural competence in LGBT health should begin during medical student and resident training so that physicians are ready to effectively care for LGBT patients upon completion of residency. Although the AAMC encourages medical schools to include sexual and gender-minority education in the curriculum, there is no official requirement.[24] A study of 150 US and Canadian medical schools revealed that LGBT-specific content was taught for a median of 5 hours, with about a third reporting 0 hours of instruction on the topic.[29] Another study demonstrated that less than half of medical students discuss patients' sexual orientation or same-sex behaviors, with 28% stating that they were apprehensive about discussing LGBT-specific health needs.[30] To address the lack of sexual health education, a multidisciplinary committee developed 20 sexual health competencies that build upon the AAMC's core competencies to facilitate the integration of LGBT education into medical school curricula.[31]

Similar to the AAMC, the Accreditation Council on Graduate Medical Education (ACGME) does not have specific educational requirements for sexual and gender minority issues for residency programs.[32] Previous work has shown that trainees do not feel comfortable caring for LGBT patients,[33] not feel comfortable taking sexual histories in LGBT patients,[34] and do not feel up-to-date on transgender screening guidelines.[35]

In addition, certain surgical specialties relevant in transgender health, including urology, obstetrics/gynecology, and plastic surgery, do not have an ACGME case log requirement for transgender patients.[36] Urology and plastic surgery residencies only provide about 1 hour of didactic exposure and 2 hours of clinical exposure in transgender patient care per year on average.[37] Surveys of plastic surgery residents/fellows, urology residents, and otolaryngology residents revealed that 64%, 54%, and 30%, respectively, were exposed to transgender patient care during residency, either through providing direct care or through didactics/education.[38–40] The Council on Resident Education in Obstetrics and Gynecology developed specific objectives for transgender patient care, but they are mainly met through readings and lectures rather than patient care.[41]

Given the need for increased LGBT health education, numerous studies have investigated the efficacy of an LGBT-specific health curriculum/intervention.[42–46] They demonstrated increased knowledge regarding LGBT health, confidence in guiding/counseling LGBT patients, and comfort in caring for LGBT patients,[42,44–46] although the changes were not retained over time in 1 study.[44]

Overall, LGBT health training in residency programs remains suboptimal. A review of the American Academy of Dermatology (AAD)'s online Basic Dermatology Curriculum revealed that only 1 of 293 (0.3%) patient cases discussed an LGBT patient: a woman in a same-sex marriage with a basal cell carcinoma.[47] An ACGME curricular mandate on LGBT health could be an effective method to integrate LGBT-specific patient care into residency curriculums.[36–39] As a specialty committed to diversity and cultural competence, dermatology training programs need not wait for a mandate to identify educational gaps in training and implement initiatives to advance the level of competence.

WHERE TO BEGIN

The first step in achieving excellence in LGBT training in your program is taking an assessment of your program's current strengths, weaknesses, and opportunities. There are various aspects to consider when assessing a residency program for LGBT culturally competent education and care. As with other aspects of resident education, the goal is to train residents in culturally competent care of LGBT patients by providing them with didactics as well as experiential training. Your program may already have a faculty member with experience or expertise in LGBT issues who can serve as an LGBT champion for the department.

Even without experience, a faculty member enthusiastic to expand their knowledge and gain expertise can be equally beneficial. Most programs can also benefit from resources outside the department. Many institutions have individuals well-versed in LGBT competency that can provide support and guidance through the process. It may also be beneficial to reach out to LGBT experts in other departments. In assessing a program, answering the following questions can help determine goals for improvement: Where (if at all) does LGBT education exist in the current curriculum? How is LGBT education currently delivered: didactics, patient encounters, surgical exercises? What opportunities can members (faculty, residents, staff) of the department identify to add LGBT education to the current curriculum? How is the department currently delivering care to meet the needs of LGBT patients (patient experience, staff training, and so forth)? What LGBT resources are available inside and outside the department?

The 2 primary goals when developing LGBT training in a residency program are curricular modifications and departmental, and perhaps institutional, climate optimization. Integration of LGBT education into the curriculum is a task for the program director, working closely with any faculty champions. Instituting departmental climate change requires collaboration and support from the department chair, because it will involve training and education of all staff in the department and may also require improvements in the processes of health care delivery in the department. To address both of these goals, the AAMC developed a resource to help guide medical educators in the process.[24]

ENHANCING THE CURRICULUM

The foundation of LGBT excellence for a dermatology department should begin with establishing fundamental knowledge of LGBT cultural competence.[48,49] The terminology specific to the care of LGBT patients can be complex and confusing. An understanding of these terms and how to approach them when interacting with patients is paramount to providing optimal care.[50] Establishing this knowledge in the department can be achieved through a didactic session involving a combination of lecture, discussion, and question and answer.[24] Ideally, faculty, residents, and staff should all be included, because this information pertains to all those in the department who interact with patients. This component of LGBT education is essential for any program because it provides the framework for culturally competent care.[50] Dermatology residents prefer active learning

methods rather than passive ones for successful learning,[51,52] and LGBT health curricula that utilize active learning have been successful.[53] Online curricula have also been developed and may present a more flexible option for additional instruction.[54]

The ACGME provides a structure for the required curriculum for dermatology residents in the form of the core competencies. There are aspects of the dermatology curriculum that present opportunities to incorporate LGBT teaching in each of the competencies. Training programs are required by the ACGME to include instruction dedicated to ethics, and issues surrounding LGBT patients, their interactions with the health care system, and disparities provide content for this education. For example, the ethics section of the *Journal of the American Academy of Dermatology* has already featured articles addressing the prescribing of isotretinoin in transgender patients[55] as well as noninvasive, reversible gender-affirming procedures in transgender adolescents.[56] In the areas of medical knowledge and patient care, gender-affirming procedures can be incorporated with the training of aesthetics and cosmetic procedures, because they highlight these principles. Involving transgender patients in resident practical sessions is an opportunity to not only provide excellent aesthetic training for residents but also have a profound impact on the lives of this marginalized patient population. Interpersonal and communication skills and practice-based learning and improvement can include the elicitation of a sexual history in a culturally competent manner to identify knowledge gaps in the appropriate screening for sexually transmitted infections based on risk factors.[50]

There are several other aspects of LGBT care that involve medical knowledge, patient care, and practice-based learning and improvement. Providers should inspect the perianal and genital area of patients, such as MSM, who may be at higher risk for human papillomavirus and other STDs.[14,57,58] Providers should perform skin cancer screening because prior work has shown that MSM have an increased risk for nonmelanoma skin cancer from increased indoor tanning[9] and that lesbians are less likely to pursue preventative care (such as skin examinations).[59] Transgender patients may require dermatologic care for androgenic acne resulting from hormone supplementation and for noninvasive facial remodeling treatments, such as neurotoxins and fillers.[60] Discussions of the HCD encountered by LGBT patients can facilitate teaching regarding system-based practice. The AAMC and Joint Commission reports on LGBT health education can also be used to guide development of a resident curriculum.[23,24] In addition to the planned curriculum, LGBT issues can be incorporated into resident evaluations and feedback.

The Dermatology Milestones Project established a set of milestones used to measure the progress of dermatology residents in achieving competence during their training. The milestones are not intended to be used directly as evaluation tools, relying on programs to develop assessment tools that correspond to the milestones. One of these milestones, Professionalism 3, specifically addresses treating patients with respect regardless of gender or sexual orientation.[61] Although the other milestones do not make specific reference to LGBT patients, these issues do fall under the broader goals of the milestones and can be incorporated in assessment tools. For example, Medical Knowledge 3 Milestone asks educators to assess residents' knowledge of the concepts and principles of noninvasive cosmetic procedures. Undeniably, there is no better metric of a dermatologist's knowledge of the principles of the aesthetic appearance than those required in the transformation accomplished with gender reassignment.[62]

Building LGBT education into the curriculum solidifies a place of importance and value and a structure for its delivery. In addition to curricular changes, departmental climate changes allow the lessons learned to be translated into excellence in caring for the dermatologic needs of the LGBT community.

ENHANCING THE CLIMATE

The Gay and Lesbian Medical Association has published a guide for enhancing the climate for LGBT students and employees that contains valuable recommendations that can be applied to residency programs as well. This guide provides comprehensive coverage of the plethora of topics to consider in respect to LGBT learners, teachers, and staff.[63] These changes can start at the department level, with enhanced education and training for all team members involved in patient care. Providers can create a welcoming environment for LGBT patients by avoiding assumptions and using nonjudgmental language.[50] When eliciting a history, providers should ask gender identity and obtain a sexual history, which includes gender or genders of sexual partners.[50] Modification of the intake paperwork requiring completion by patients can be made more inclusive of gender and spousal/partner information.[23,64–66]

The Veterans Affairs Boston Healthcare System shared their method of increasing LGBT cultural competency at multiple levels: clinical, structural, and organizational.[67] Their model was based on the cultural competence model of Betancourt and colleagues[68] to address racial/ethnic disparities. Organizational methods included formation of a diversity committee, writing LGBT patient/provider policies, assessing readiness for change, and participation in the Healthcare Equity Index. Structural methods included promoting health education and empowering staff and patients. Clinical methods included training providers at orientation and providing continuing education and participation at conferences and creating local patient support groups.[67]

Although provider or system-level changes are beneficial, organizational changes are ultimately necessary in optimizing LGBT health care.[69] An LGBT champion in your department may be afforded to opportunity to serve a similar role more broadly at your institution. Eckstrand and colleagues[69] highlight several key elements that could reduce LGBT HCD (with potential implementation strategies): "organizational champions" (having LGBT providers and students as well as educational innovators), "organizational priority" (institutional LGBT diversity and inclusion), "depth of mission" (LGBT inclusion in mission/philosophy, LGBT training for new hires, and LGBT-inclusive CME requirements), "commitment to continuous learning" (teaching LGBT-specific health needs with training opportunities), "commitment to diversity and inclusion" (recruiting LGBT staff, track LGBT outcomes, celebrate LGBT events), and "organizational resources" (funding and support for LGBT health activities and research). Although it is an untested framework that was derived from existing models to address racial/ethnic/sex HCD,[69] it provides a conceptual framework for how to implement and assess improvement.

SHARING YOUR EXCELLENCE IN LESBIAN, GAY, BISEXUAL, AND TRANSGENDER CARE

Once you have created a climate of cultural competence for LGBT health care in your department, you should not hesitate to publicize your efforts to this vulnerable patient population. Choosing a physician is an incredibly difficult task for LGBT patient because there are limited means to determine a provider's sensitivity to issues specific to this population.[70,71] To that end, the Gay and Lesbian Medical Association maintains a directory of providers who attest their commitment to cultural competence regarding the LGBT community. The efforts to incorporate LGBT training and sensitivity in your residency program place your program in the forefront of the wave of progress in the field and more than justify your inclusion in this provider list. Reaching out to other clinics already providing culturally competent care can establish a referral network for LGBT patients.

ADDITIONAL RESOURCES

In addition to those mentioned previously, there are resources within the specialty of dermatology that can provide support and guidance in incorporating LGBT training into your program. The Gay and Lesbian Dermatology Association includes the promotion and dissemination of LGBT education in its mission as well as providing a mentorship program to promote the development and advancement leaders with interest in LGBT health care. The organization also maintains a network of dermatologists capable of providing valuable insight into the LGBT training process. In recognizing the value of considering LGBT issues in dermatology, the AAD has developed an LGBT expert resource group. The AAD can help connect you with members of this group, all of whom have a dedication to advancing LGBT care in dermatology and are eager and enthusiastic to provide support.

SUMMARY

LGBT patients face significant health care difficulties and disparities. Addressing these challenges through enhancing dermatology training programs will build the foundation for improvement. Although there are aspects of LGBT education that are serious in nature, do not lose sight of the fact that there are many other elements that can be incredibly fun. There is no one more qualified to teach the aesthetics of the male and female face than a drag queen who understands facial contours with enough knowledge to transform their appearance. The lesson will be easy to learn from an experienced entertainer cracking jokes all the way. They may also serve as an invaluable resource for learning camouflaging techniques that translate to issues beyond the LGBT realm, such as vitiligo. The recommendations in this article serve as a guide for incorporating LGBT issues into a dermatology residency training program.

DISCLOSURE

The authors have nothing to disclose.

REFERENCES

1. Gates GJ. LGBT demographics: comparisons among population-based surveys. The Williams Institute, UCLA School of Law; 2017. Available at: http://williamsinstitute.law.ucla.edu/wp-content/uploads/lgbt-demogs-sep-2014.pdf. Accessed March 20, 2019.
2. Office of Disease Prevention and Health Promotion. Lesbian, gay, bisexual, and transgender health. Healthy people 2020. Available at: https://www.healthypeople.gov/2020/topics-objectives/topic/lesbian-gay-bisexual-and-transgender-health. Accessed March 20, 2019.
3. Hafeez H, Zeshan M, Tahir MA, et al. Health care disparities among lesbian, gay, bisexual, and transgender youth: a literature review. Cureus 2017;9(4):e1184.
4. Institute of Medicine (US) Committee on Lesbian, Gay, Bisexual, and Transgender Health Issues and Research Gaps and Opportunities. The health of lesbian, gay, bisexual, and transgender people: building a foundation for better understanding 2011. Washington (DC). Available at: https://www.ncbi.nlm.nih.gov/books/NBK64806/. Accessed March 20, 2019.
5. Liszewski W, Peebles JK, Yeung H, et al. Persons of nonbinary gender–awareness, visibility, and health disparities. N Engl J Med 2018;379(25):2391–3.
6. Meyer IH. Prejudice as stress: conceptual and measurement problems. Am J Public Health 2003;93(2):262–5.
7. Rodriguez A, Agardh A, Asamoah BO. Self-reported discrimination in health-care settings based on recognizability as transgender: a cross-sectional study among transgender U.S. citizens. Arch Sex Behav 2018;47(4):973–85.
8. Understanding the health needs of LGBT people, March 2016. Available at: https://www.lgbthealtheducation.org/wp-content/uploads/LGBTHealthDisparitiesMar2016.pdf. Accessed March 20, 2019.
9. Mansh M, Katz KA, Linos E, et al. Association of skin cancer and indoor tanning in sexual minority men and women. JAMA Dermatol 2015;151(12):1308–16.
10. Blashill AJ, Safren SA. Skin cancer risk behaviors among US men: the role of sexual orientation. Am J Public Health 2014;104(9):1640–1.
11. Coleman E, Bockting W, Botzer M, et al. Standards of care for the health of transsexual, transgender, and gender-nonconforming people, version 7. Int J Transgend 2012;13(4):165–232.
12. Mundluru SN, Larson AR. Medical dermatologic conditions in transgender women. Int J Womens Dermatol 2018;4(4):212–5.
13. Baral SD, Poteat T, Stromdahl S, et al. Worldwide burden of HIV in transgender women: a systematic review and meta-analysis. Lancet Infect Dis 2013;13(3):214–22.
14. Schofield AM, Sadler L, Nelson L, et al. A prospective study of anal cancer screening in

HIV-positive and negative MSM. AIDS 2016;30(9): 1375–83.

15. Colon-Lopez V, Shiels MS, Machin M, et al. Anal cancer risk among people with HIV infection in the United States. J Clin Oncol 2018;36(1):68–75.

16. D'Souza G, Wentz A, Wiley D, et al. Anal cancer screening in men who have sex with men in the multicenter AIDS Cohort Study. J Acquir Immune Defic Syndr 2016;71(5):570–6.

17. Boos MD, Ginsberg BA, Peebles JK. Prescribing isotretinoin for transgender youth: a pledge for more inclusive care. Pediatr Dermatol 2019;36(1): 169–71.

18. Campos-Munoz L, Lopez-De Lara D, Rodriguez-Rojo ML, et al. Transgender adolescents and acne: a cases series. Pediatr Dermatol 2018; 35(3):e155–8.

19. Katz KA. Transgender patients, isotretinoin, and US Food and Drug Administration-mandated risk evaluation and mitigation strategies: a prescription for inclusion. JAMA Dermatol 2016;152(5):513–4.

20. Motosko CC, Zakhem GA, Pomeranz MK, et al. Acne: a side-effect of masculinizing hormonal therapy in transgender patients. Br J Dermatol 2019; 180(1):26–30.

21. Trinh MH, Agenor M, Austin SB, et al. Health and healthcare disparities among U.S. women and men at the intersection of sexual orientation and race/ethnicity: a nationally representative cross-sectional study. BMC Public Health 2017;17(1):964.

22. Meyer IH. Prejudice, social stress, and mental health in lesbian, gay, and bisexual populations: conceptual issues and research evidence. Psychol Bull 2003;129(5):674–97.

23. The Joint Commission. Advancing effective communication, cultural competence, and patient- and family centered care for the lesbian, gay, bisexual, and transgender (LGBT) community: a field guide 2011. Oak Brook (IL), Available at: https://www.jointcommission.org/assets/1/18/LGBT FieldGuide.pdf. Accessed March 20, 2019.

24. Association of American Medical Colleges (AAMC). Implementing curricular and institutional climate changes to improve health care for individuals who are LGBT, gender nonconforming, or born with DSD: a resource for medical educators. In: Hollenbach AD, Eckstrand KL, Dreger A, editors. Association of American Medical Colleges. 2014. Available at: https://members.aamc.org/eweb/upload/Executive %20LGBT%20FINAL.pdf 2014. Accessed March 20, 2019.

25. Daniel H, Butkus R. Health and Public Policy Committee of American College of Physicians. Lesbian, gay, bisexual, and transgender health disparities: executive summary of a policy position paper from the American College of Physicians. Ann Intern Med 2015;163:135–7.

26. National Institutes of Health Sexual and Gender Minority Research Coordinating Committee website. NIH FY 2016-2020 strategic plan to advance research on the health and well-being of sexual and gender minorities. Available at: https://dpcpsi.nih. gov/sites/default/files/sgmStrategicPlan.pdf. Accessed March 25, 2019.

27. Bachmann LH, Grimley DM, Gao H, et al. Impact of a computer-assisted, provider-delivered intervention on sexual risk behaviors in HIV-positive men who have sex with men (MSM) in a primary care setting. AIDS Educ Prev 2013;25(2):87–101.

28. Patel P, Bush T, Mayer K, et al. Routine brief risk-reduction counseling with biannual STD testing reduces STD incidence among HIV-infected men who have sex with men in care. Sex Transm Dis 2012;39(6):470–4.

29. Obedin-Maliver J, Goldsmith ES, Stewart L, et al. Lesbian, gay, bisexual, and transgender-related content in undergraduate medical education. JAMA 2011;306(9):971–7.

30. Sanchez NF, Rabatin J, Sanchez JP, et al. Medical students' ability to care for lesbian, gay, bisexual, and transgendered patients. Fam Med 2006;38(1): 21–7.

31. Bayer CR, Eckstrand KL, Knudson G, et al. Sexual health competencies for undergraduate medical education in North America. J Sex Med 2017;14(4): 535–40.

32. Accreditation Council for Graduate Medical Education. ACGME program requirements for graduate medical education in internal medicine 2017. Available at: http://www.acgme.org/Portals/0/PFAssets/ ProgramRequirements/140_internal_medicine_2017-07-01.pdf?ver=2017-06-30-083345-723. Accessed March 20, 2019.

33. Honigberg MC, Eshel N, Luskin MR, et al. Curricular time, patient exposure, and comfort caring for lesbian, gay, bisexual, and transgender patients among recent medical graduates. LGBT Health 2017;4(3):237–9.

34. Hayes V, Blondeau W, Bing-You RG. Assessment of medical student and resident/fellow knowledge, comfort, and training with sexual history taking in LGBTQ patients. Fam Med 2015;47(5):383–7.

35. Johnston CD, Shearer LS. Internal medicine resident attitudes, prior education, comfort, and knowledge regarding delivering comprehensive primary care to transgender patients. Transgend Health 2017; 2(1):91–5.

36. Morrison SD, Wilson SC, Smith JR. Are we adequately preparing our trainees to care for transgender patients? J Grad Med Educ 2017;9(2):258.

37. Morrison SD, Dy GW, Chong HJ, et al. Transgender-related education in plastic surgery and urology residency programs. J Grad Med Educ 2017;9(2): 178–83.

38. Morrison SD, Chong HJ, Dy GW, et al. Educational exposure to transgender patient care in plastic surgery training. Plast Reconstr Surg 2016;138(4): 944–53.

39. Dy GW, Osbun NC, Morrison SD, et al. Exposure to and attitudes regarding transgender education among urology residents. J Sex Med 2016;13(10): 1466–72.

40. Massenburg BM, Morrison SD, Rashidi V, et al. Educational exposure to transgender patient care in otolaryngology training. J Craniofac Surg 2018; 29(5):1252–7.

41. Grimstad FW, Satterwhite CL, Wieneke CL. Assessing residency program approaches to the transgender health CREOG objective. Transgend Health 2016;1(1):69–74.

42. Ufomata E, Eckstrand KL, Hasley P, et al. Comprehensive internal medicine residency curriculum on primary care of patients who identify as LGBT. LGBT Health 2018;5(6):375–80.

43. Streed CG Jr, Hedian HF, Bertram A, et al. Assessment of internal medicine resident preparedness to care for lesbian, gay, bisexual, transgender, and queer/questioning patients. J Gen Intern Med 2019;34(6):893–8.

44. Kidd JD, Bockting W, Cabaniss DL, et al. Special-"T" training: extended follow-up results from a residency-wide professionalism workshop on transgender health. Acad Psychiatry 2016;40(5):802–6.

45. Thomas DD, Safer JD. A simple intervention raised resident-physician willingness to assist transgender patients seeking hormone therapy. Endocr Pract 2015;21(10):1134–42.

46. McGarry KA, Clarke JG, Cyr MG, et al. Evaluating a lesbian and gay health care curriculum. Teach Learn Med 2002;14(4):244–8.

47. Park AJ, Katz KA. Paucity of lesbian, gay, bisexual, and transgender health-related content in the basic dermatology curriculum. JAMA Dermatol 2018; 154(5):614–5.

48. Butler M, McCreedy E, Schwer N, et al. Improving cultural competence to reduce health disparities 2016. Rockville (MD). Available at: https://www.ncbi.nlm.nih.gov/books/NBK361118/. Accessed March 20, 2019.

49. Baker K, Beagan B. Making assumptions, making space: an anthropological critique of cultural competency and its relevance to queer patients. Med Anthropol Q 2014;28(4):578–98.

50. Yeung H, Luk KM, Chen SC, et al. Dermatologic care for lesbian, gay, bisexual, and transgender persons: terminology, demographics, health disparities, and approaches to care. J Am Acad Dermatol 2019; 80(3):581–9.

51. Stratman EJ, Vogel CA, Reck SJ, et al. Analysis of dermatology resident self-reported successful learning styles and implications for core competency curriculum development. Med Teach 2008;30(4):420–5.

52. Stratman E, Dyer J. Problem-based learning: an approach to dermatology resident education. Arch Dermatol 2002;138(10):1299–302.

53. Klein EW, Nakhai M. Caring for LGBTQ patients: methods for improving physician cultural competence. Int J Psychiatry Med 2016;51(4):315–24.

54. Barber ME, Dresche J, Rosari V. The GAP online LGBT mental health curriculum. J Gay Lesbian Ment Health 2012;16(1):41–8.

55. Yeung H, Chen SC, Katz KA, et al. Prescribing isotretinoin in the United States for transgender individuals: ethical considerations. J Am Acad Dermatol 2016;75(3):648–51.

56. Waldman RA, Waldman SD, Grant-Kels JM. The ethics of performing noninvasive, reversible gender-affirming procedures on transgender adolescents. J Am Acad Dermatol 2018;79(6): 1166–8.

57. Katz MH, Katz KA, Bernostein KT, et al. We need data on anal screening effectiveness before focusing on increasing it. Am J Public Health 2010; 100(11):2016–7.

58. Charny JW, Kovarik CL. LGBT access to health care: a dermatologist's role in building a therapeutic relationship. Cutis 2017;99(4):228–9.

59. Conron KJ, Mimiaga MJ, Landers SJ. A population-based study of sexual orientation identity and gender differences in adult health. Am J Public Health 2010;100(10):1953–60.

60. Ginsberg BA. Dermatologic care of the transgender patient. Int J Womens Dermatol 2017;3(1):65–7.

61. The dermatology milestone project. J Grad Med Educ 2014;6(1 Suppl 1):47–70.

62. Dhingra N, Bonati LM, Wang EB, et al. Medical and aesthetic procedural dermatology recommendations for transgender patients undergoing transition. J Am Acad Dermatol 2019;80(6):1712–21.

63. Snowdon S. Recommendations for enhancing the climate for LGBT students and employees in health professional schools: a GLMA white paper. Washington, DC: GLMA; 2013. Available at: http://www.glma.org/_data/n_0001/resources/live/Recommendations%20for%20Enhancing%20LGBT%20Climate%20in%20Health%20Professional%20Schools.pdf. Accessed March 30, 2019.

64. Ard KL, Makadon HJ. Improving the health care of lesbian, gay, bisexual and transgender people: understanding and eliminating health disparities. Boston: The Fenway Institute. Available at: https://www.lgbthealtheducation.org/wp-content/uploads/Improving-the-Health-of-LGBT-People.pdf. Accessed March 30, 2019.

65. Gay & Lesbian Medical Association. Guidelines for care of lesbian, gay, bisexual, and transgender patients. Available at: http://glma.org/_data/n_0001/

resources/live/GLMA%20guidelines%202006%20 FINAL.pdf. Accessed March 30, 2019.

66. Coren JS, Coren CM, Pagliaro SN, et al. Assessing your office for care of lesbian, gay, bisexual, and transgender patients. Health Care Manag (Frederick) 2011;30(1):66–70.

67. Ruben MA, Shipherd JC, Topor D, et al. Advancing LGBT health care policies and clinical care within a large academic health care system: a case study. J Homosex 2017;64(10):1411–31.

68. Betancourt JR, Green AR, Carrillo JE, et al. Defining cultural competence: a practical framework for addressing racial/ethnic disparities in health and health care. Public Health Rep 2003;118(4): 293–302.

69. Eckstrand KL, Lunn MR, Yehia BR. Applying organizational change to promote lesbian, gay, bisexual, and transgender inclusion and reduce health disparities. LGBT Health 2017;4(3):174–80.

70. Jann JT, Edmiston EK, Ehrenfeld JM. Important considerations for addressing LGBT health care competency. Am J Public Health 2015;105(11):e8.

71. Khalili J, Leung LB, Diamant AL. Finding the perfect doctor: identifying lesbian, gay, bisexual, and transgender-competent physicians. Am J Public Health 2015;105(6):1114–9.

Moving?

Make sure your subscription moves with you!

To notify us of your new address, find your **Clinics Account Number** (located on your mailing label above your name), and contact customer service at:

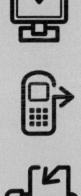

Email: journalscustomerservice-usa@elsevier.com

800-654-2452 (subscribers in the U.S. & Canada)
314-447-8871 (subscribers outside of the U.S. & Canada)

Fax number: 314-447-8029

Elsevier Health Sciences Division
Subscription Customer Service
3251 Riverport Lane
Maryland Heights, MO 63043

ELSEVIER

Moving?

Make sure your subscription moves with you!

To notify us of your new address, find your Clinics Account Number (located on your mailing label above your name), and contact customer service at:

Email: journalscustomerservice-usa@elsevier.com

800-654-2452 (subscribers in the U.S. & Canada)
314-447-8871 (subscribers outside of the U.S. & Canada)

Fax number: 314-447-8029

Elsevier Health Sciences Division
Subscription Customer Service
3251 Riverport Lane
Maryland Heights, MO 63043

To ensure uninterrupted delivery of your subscription, please notify us at least 4 weeks in advance of move.

Printed and bound by CPI Group (UK) Ltd, Croydon, CR0 4YY

03/10/2024

01040307-0011